Exploding the Make-up Myth

for all women over **25**

NOUK TAYLER-VIEIRA

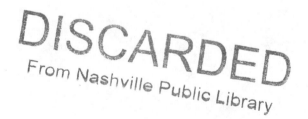
SALLY MILNER PUBLISHING

First published in 1992 by
Sally Milner Publishing Pty Ltd
67 Glassop Street
Birchgrove NSW 2041 Australia

© Nouk Tayler-Vieira, 1992

Production by Sylvana Scannapiego,
Island Graphics
Design by Diana Kureen
Illustrations by Howard Hook
Photography by Rob Cooper
Typeset in Australia by Asset Typesetting Pty Ltd
Printed in Australia by Impact Printing

National Library of Australia
Cataloguing-in-Publication data:

Tayler-Vieira, Nouk
    Exploding the make-up myth.

    Includes index.
    ISBN 1 86351 073 7.

    1. Cosmetics. 2. Beauty, Personal. I. Title.

646.72

Contents

ACKNOWLEDGEMENTS

I want to thank these loving and supportive people who have made this
book a reality:

Rob Cooper, for his expertise and patience while producing such
wonderful photos.

Howard Hook, for such precise and descriptive illustrations.

The models in this book, all of whom volunteered their time and assistance.
They are all everyday women with 'full on' lives — thank you.

Sally Milner, for her faith and determination.

Margaret Falk, for endless nights of editing before the book went to the publisher.

Cheryl Doolan, for her dependable assistance during difficult times.

Evelyne Tayler, my mother and a wonderful skin beauty specialist, Chic et Belle,
Cairns, for her loving support.

Tom Vieira, my soul mate, without whom none of this book would have been
conceived. Thank you for believing in me.

DEDICATION

Do you know how this book came about?

Every woman that has come to me for make-up advice over the years has learned much from me, but I have gained so much more from them in return.

It is to these wonderful women that I dedicate this book.

Without their constant search for a 'better way', I would not have been driven to find the answer ... thank you.

A letter
from the author

*H*ello, and welcome to you, the woman over 25, who wants to explode the make-up myth and capture the previously elusive art of enhancing your own natural beauty. This book is for you. The level of success it can help you achieve depends upon understanding my reasons for writing it.

Naturally, there are basic facts and theories, methods and techniques of make-up to convey. Also, I have an attitude to express about individuals, beauty and positive thinking, and a belief that together, you and I can do better than the advertising manipulators and cosmetic sales representatives who have other things on their minds than the way you want to look!

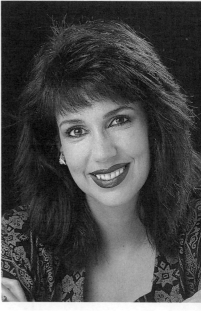

So, before we embark on this journey, I'd like you to have a mirror handy, seat yourself in good natural lighting, and prepare yourself for a voyage of personal discovery.

Most make-up information around today is geared toward making you aware of your facial flaws and telling you how to disguise them. Numerous make-up products are promoted to conceal particular aspects of your face that are considered to be 'flaws'.

Not much has been done to provide you, the consumer — the wearer of these make-up products — with esteem-bolstering information such as how to identify and maximise your best features. Honestly, do you know exactly what your best features are? If you do, then you're in the minority. Most women I've talked with have known more about their so-called flaws or faults than their positive features.

The success of your new make-up lies in the recognition and appreciation of your facial features, and not in your flaws.

The reason the models in this book look so great in their 'after' shots is because I concentrated on their best features. For example, look at Plate 2, page 13; Plate 4, page 17; Plate 8, page 23; Plate 10, page 25; and Plate 12, page 27.

As you will see, these women all look individual, vibrant and naturally beautiful. There is no 'nose shading' or clever contouring to alter their facial shapes. Unlike most before and after photos, no photographic tricks such as special-effect lighting, soft-focus lenses or 'touch-up' techniques (to eradicate lines, wrinkles and shadows) have been used. These photos are true to life, and the women I have chosen are aged between 25 and 60 years old. I've worked only on the positive aspects of their natural beauty. Most of the women who've been to see me for make-up advice believe they are lacking in some aspect of facial beauty. Various features such as noses, mouths and face shapes are so often cited as a problem. It seems as if many women are just not happy with the features with which they were born.

The appearance of wrinkles, lines and sagging skin as we grow older seems to be another cause of dismay. Nobody likes the physical aspects of the ageing process, do they? If you are unhappy about your facial features or the effects of ageing, I believe you have one of three choices to make.

1 Accept and appreciate what you have (and you'll actually become more and more beautiful).

2 Have cosmetic surgery (that is, 'corrective' surgery or a face lift).

3 Resent your face (and never be happy).

I personally believe that the first choice is the best, while the second can be an option. The third won't really get you anywhere, except older and less attractive as time goes by. In my view, every woman is naturally beautiful, regardless of age. The only thing preventing you from seeing your own beauty is your attitude.

Every woman has the potential to be beautiful in her own way, whatever her age. Beauty has no age barrier. The real secret is learning to appreciate yourself. This means changing your way of thinking about yourself.

If you have been telling yourself that your face isn't beautiful, you'll probably believe it by now, such is the power of thought. So if you really want to be beautiful, the change is there waiting for you. Change your attitude of mind by using positive affirmations such as this one:

"I am uniquely beautiful, and I'm at a beautiful age in my life."

Positive affirmations are powerful tools which will help you grow and discover a beauty which is yours and yours alone.

If you really want to see your true beauty, you must practise your affirmations. Make one up if you like. Say it to yourself at least three times a day. Remember, an affirmation must always be said in the present tense: "I am now beautiful", not "I will be beautiful".

A positive attitude, coupled with the vital make-up knowledge in this book, will help you look, feel and know just how individually beautiful you are!

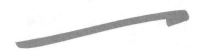

Introduction
let's study art

Have you ever been given confusing or conflicting advice on make-up, or read books written by Hollywood make-up artists who use 'perfect', young models, and tell you that you can achieve the same look? Have you bought the new season's make-up colours because advertising suggests that this is your only avenue to staying young and attractive.

If your answer is 'yes' to any or all of the above questions, and you are dissatisfied, then you deserve to read this book. After researching thousands of women mostly over the age of 25, the response I've had to these questions has been a resounding 'yes'. Women are dissatisfied with the information that's available and, in most cases, are unhappy with the make-up that they have purchased.

This book should clear up the confusion and the fear of the unknown about make-up. The secret to a youthful, attractive and natural make-up is very simple. I know it sounds unbelievable but it's true.

A car has a blind spot — obvious, and yet out of sight. Make-up, too, has its blind spot. After teaching more than 4500 women, I have found very few women know or understand that make-up is an art. It is no exaggeration to say it is an artform, to which the principles of art always apply. Simple? Yes! And yet make-up has seldom been taught using these principles.

The principles, or 'keys' as I prefer to call them, of art are:

1 Colour.

2 Balance.

3 Light and shade.

This book is founded upon these three keys. It will help you separate the 'art' from the confusion of fashion and beauty fads. You will notice that there are no photographs using young, 'perfect' models, no trick photography or special effects.

This is a book about the everyday woman, lines and all!

This is a book about you.

It is dedicated to you.

It is for you!

It will help you discover your unique beauty and show you how to bring it out.

It will free you from the need to slavishly follow fashion.

It will liberate you and help you to be the individual you are.

You are beautiful already, with natural assets. I will show you how to accentuate that beauty and maintain a natural, younger appearance.

Once you understand the principles of light, shade, colour and balance, you will know which colours suit you and how to apply them once and for all!

The Keys

whose advice should you take?

I'd like you to select one of the following two statements; the one with which you feel most comfortable.

CHOICE 1

Would you like to be totally colour co-ordinated and fashionable, using only the latest fashion make-up shades and trends — even though these may age you by as much as five to 10 years?

CHOICE 2

Would you prefer to look five to 10 years younger, sporting your individual make-up style as attractively as possible, while using a set selection and application of colours?

If you chose the first option, the advertising world has won you. But please read on. You may change your mind. If you chose the second option, then you are one of the millions of women seeking the truth about make-up.

Over the years, you've probably spent many hundreds of dollars on make-up, possibly realising that a large percentage of your purchases rarely, if ever, get used. Why?

◢ Did you receive advice?

◢ Advice on what colours to buy?

◢ Advice on their applications?

This advice may have come from 'professional' sources. Such as:

◢ Sales consultants.

◢ Make-up books by Hollywood make-up artists, rather than books for the everyday woman.

◢ Make-up books sponsored by cosmetic companies to promote their products.

◢ Magazines.

If your information has been gathered from any of the above sources, then you must ask yourself, "What is their chief motivation?" Is it to assist you in both the selection and application of your make-up, or is it to sell a product?

Most of the make-up information you'll receive from these sources will either be confusing or contradictory. This is because the cosmetic industry's primary objective is sales; sales to you, the consumer. Education is not on the agenda! And, for as long as the world of make-up is fuelled by fashion and beauty fads, it will continue to be shrouded in mystery and confusion, especially for the everyday woman.

The more ignorant of the art of make-up you remain, the more influenced by fashion and advertising you'll be. Free yourself from this stranglehold!

If you have a colour magazine with a cosmetic advertisement in it, open it to 'one of those ads' right now. Are you tempted to buy the make-up product advertised because you can see how great it looks on the model? Before you seriously entertain the thought of purchasing this particular product, ask yourself a few questions:

▰ Is the model close to your age?

▰ Is she young and near-perfect?

▰ Have clever photographic tricks such as diffused lighting and soft-focus lenses been used? And, to remove any remaining imperfections, is special-effects film processing in evidence?

No wonder she looks perfect!

Given access to the same photographic resources, no matter what your age you could also look sensational — real covergirl material. For an example of photographic ingenuity at work, look at Janelle in Figs 1, 2 and 3 on pages 8-9. In Fig 2, her make-up is incorrect. In Fig 1, she has the correct make-up application. Now look at Fig 3 and study the differences. All skin imperfections including lines and wrinkles have been removed. This process is

called a 'face-job' (touch-up) and is used commonly in professional cosmetic-advertising photographs. Interesting, isn't it?

Make-up advertising owes its success more to photographic techniques than to the actual product being promoted. The same can be said of the 'beauty' of film stars on film. Special conditions and the use of soft-focus lenses or body-doubles are common effects in creating an illusion.

Seeking commercially biased advice is clearly not to your advantage. Learning about your make-up is. So, how do you free yourself from the stranglehold of cosmetic advertising? By make-up education. By learning the art of make-up.

THE ART OF THE FACE

Those of you who chose the second answer on page 6 and those of you who ultimately want to look fresher, younger and more of an individual deserve to know the keys to make-up. These keys are paramount, at any age, when selecting and producing a personalised

OVERPAGE: *A photographic touch-up job.*

Fig 1. Photograph of Janelle with correctly applied make-up.

Fig 2. Janelle with incorrectly applied make-up.

Fig 3. The results of a photographic touch-up job on an identical photograph to the one in Figure 1.

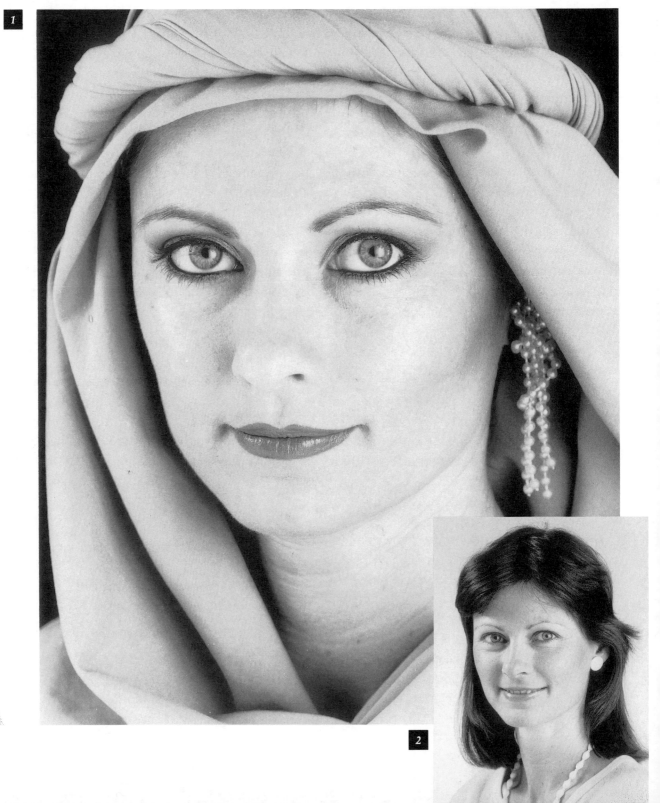

1

2

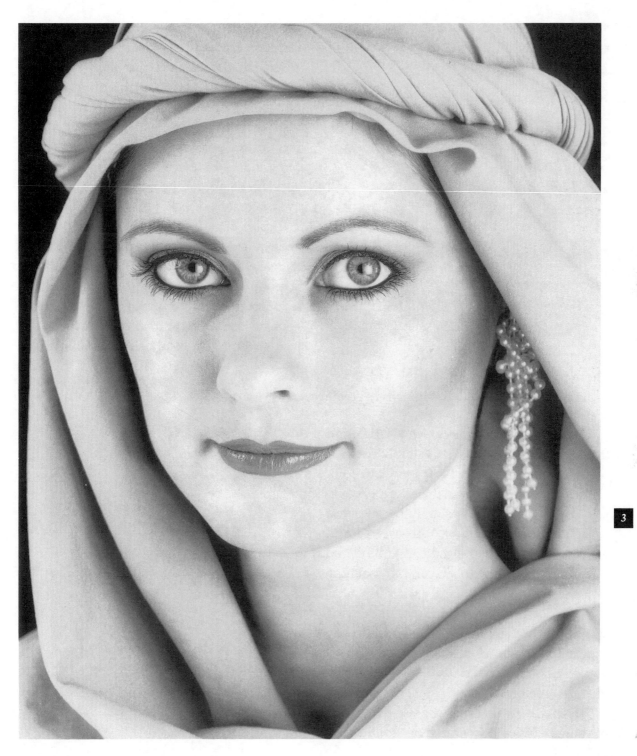

3

9

make-up. They are based on the proven principles of art, and comprise:

1 *Colour*

2 *Balance*

3 *Light and shade*

These principles were explored by such artists as Michelangelo, da Vinci and Rubens to create realistic portraits.

The art of make-up is not much different from painting on canvas: it is simply painting on the face. If I were to ask you now to paint a realistic, three-dimensional landscape, could you do it? Probably not, simply because you haven't been taught how to. You haven't learnt which colours to use for the background and foreground, or how to make your painting 'come to life'.

If you don't know the principles underlying successful painting, how in the world do you expect to be able to select your best make-up colours and produce an individual make-up for your face?

Now perhaps you can recognise the source of your confusion about make-up. To illustrate the world-wide enormity of make-up confusion, consider the following example.

Fashion has dictated that blue eyeshadow (preferably frosted) be the number one, bestselling colour in the world today. In truth, it is the most harsh and ageing of all the colours available. If frosted, it will accentuate lines and wrinkles (even if none is normally apparent) and overpower the beauty of the eyes themselves.

This is a perfect example of how women need to be released from the present world of make-up ignorance. So, get ready. This is a lesson — a very simple lesson — taught to help create a more individual, fresher and younger you. It is but one of the many easily learnt lessons that comprise the Art of the Face.

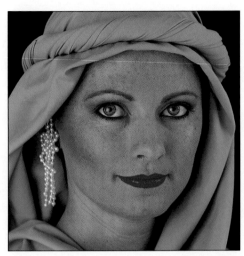

See how it works

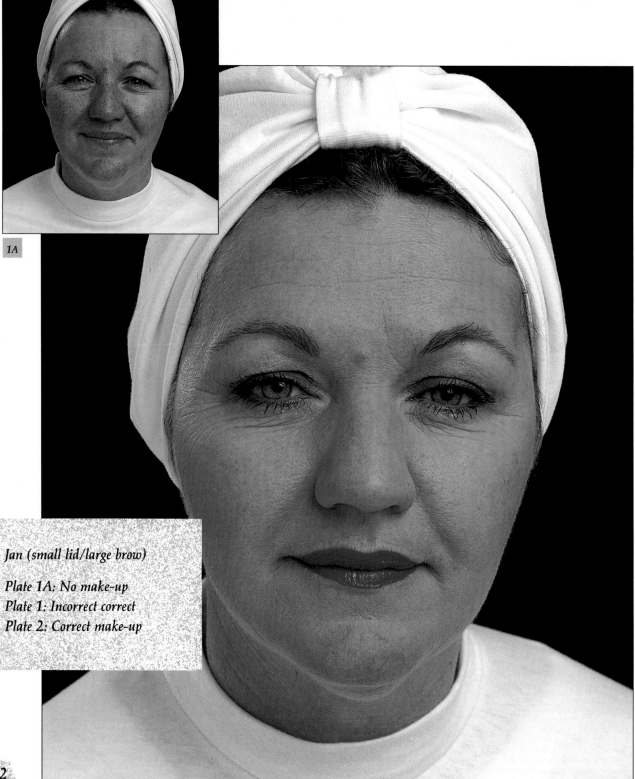

1A

Jan (small lid/large brow)

Plate 1A: No make-up
Plate 1: Incorrect correct
Plate 2: Correct make-up

12

1

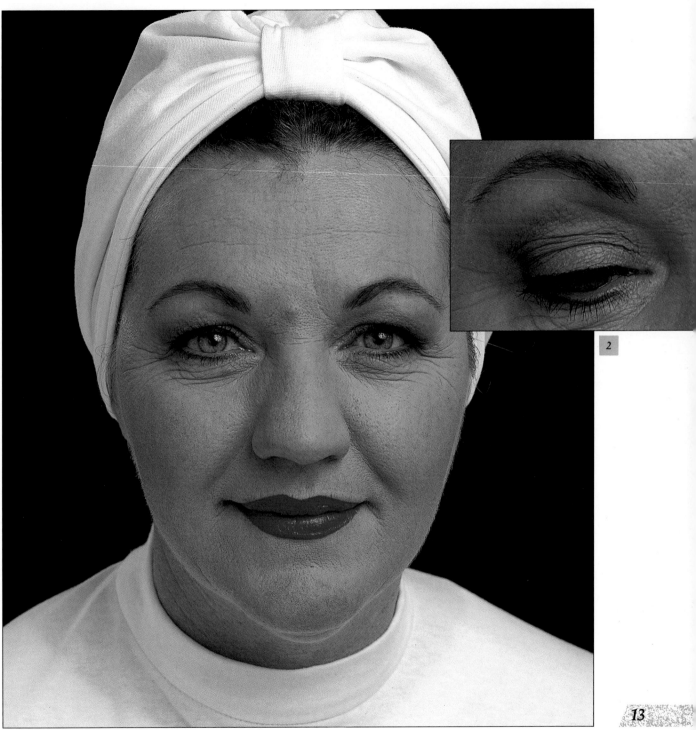

2

13

The Decorative Eyeshadow

AGEING COLOURS

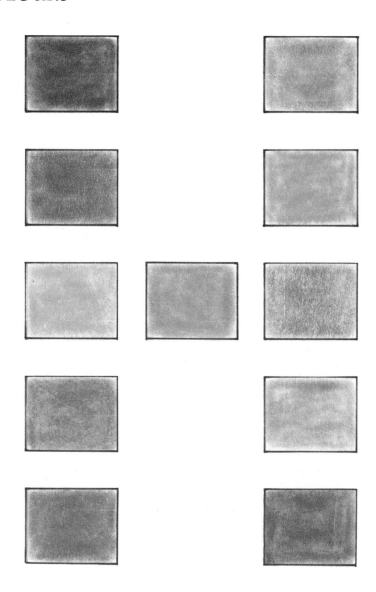

Colours

"USELESS" MEDIUM INTENSITY COLOURS

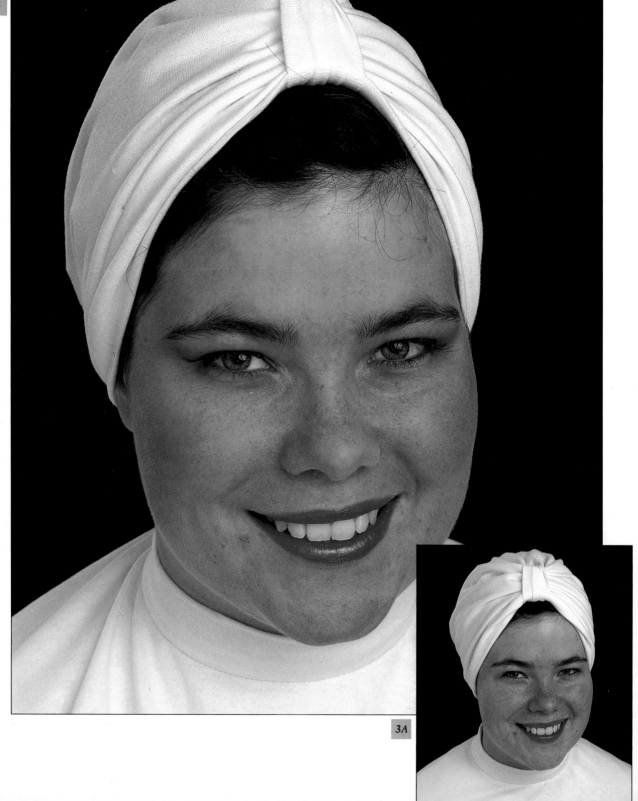

3A

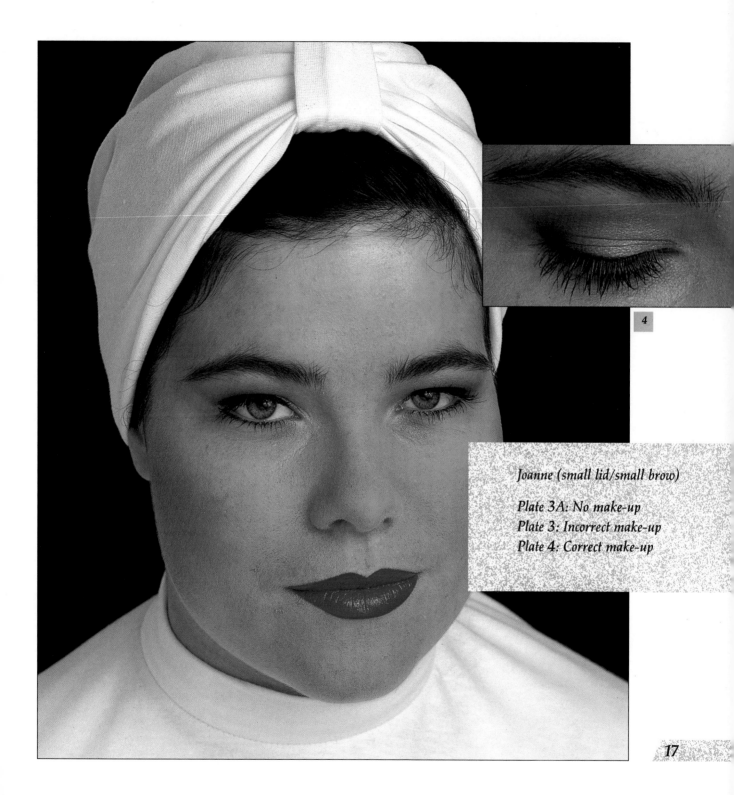

Joanne (small lid/small brow)

Plate 3A: No make-up
Plate 3: Incorrect make-up
Plate 4: Correct make-up

4

17

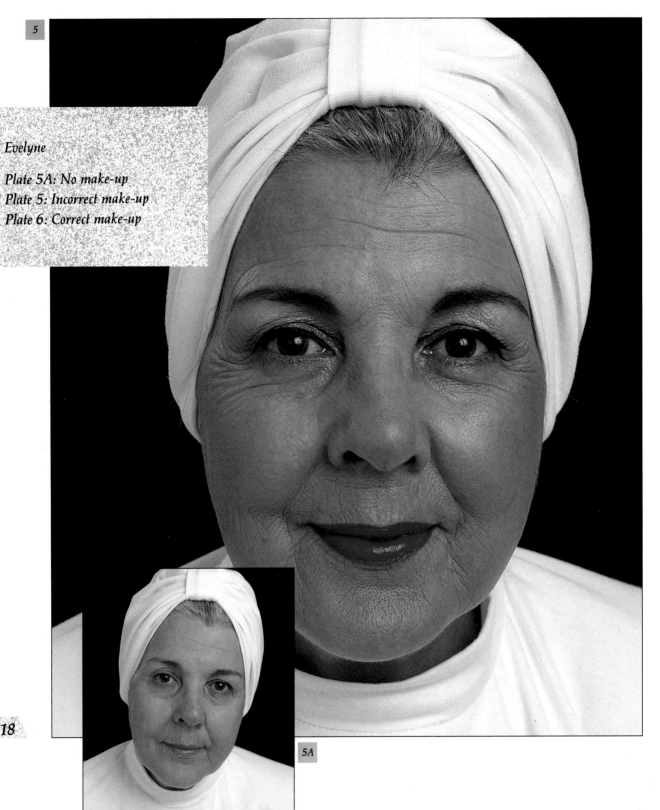

5

Evelyne

Plate 5A: No make-up
Plate 5: Incorrect make-up
Plate 6: Correct make-up

18

5A

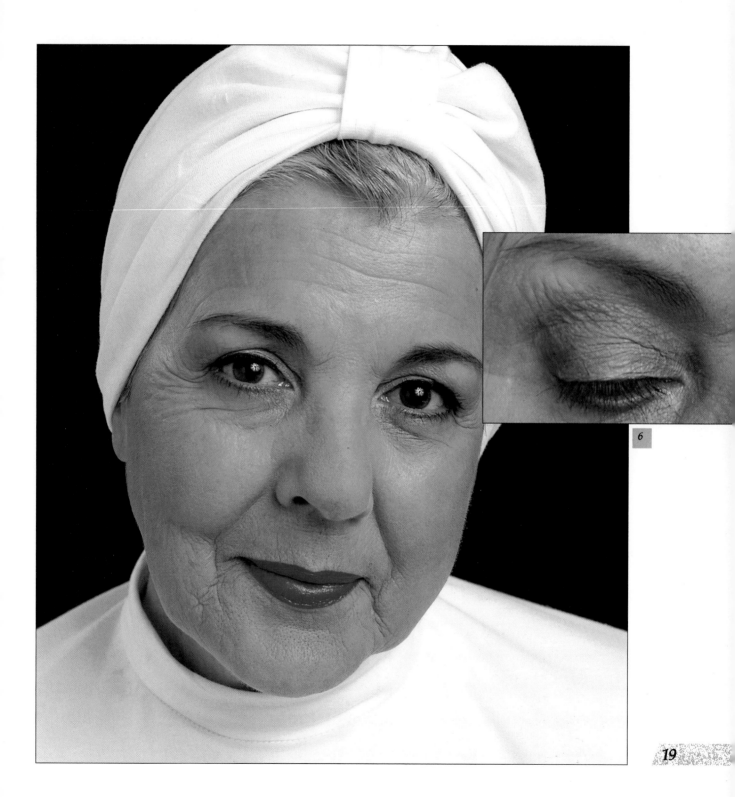

6

19

The Natural Compatible C...

eyeshadow colour chart

LIGHT SHADOWS

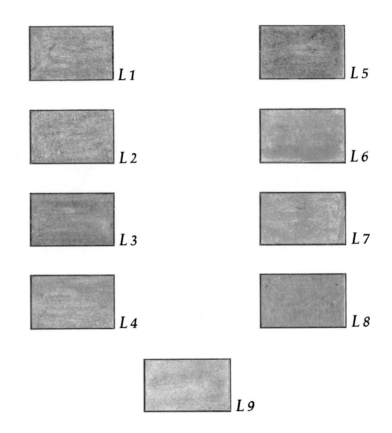

L 1

L 2

L 3

L 4

L 5

L 6

L 7

L 8

L 9

BLUSH SHADOW

BL 1

ours

DEEP SHADOWS

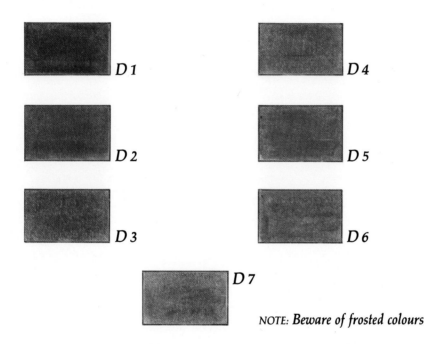

D 1

D 4

D 2

D 5

D 3

D 6

D 7

NOTE: *Beware of frosted colours*

SHADOW LINERS

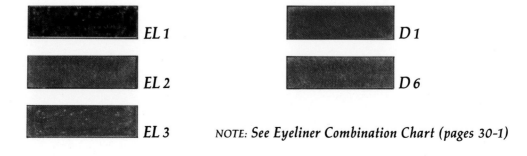

EL 1

EL 2

EL 3

D 1

D 6

NOTE: *See Eyeliner Combination Chart (pages 30-1)*

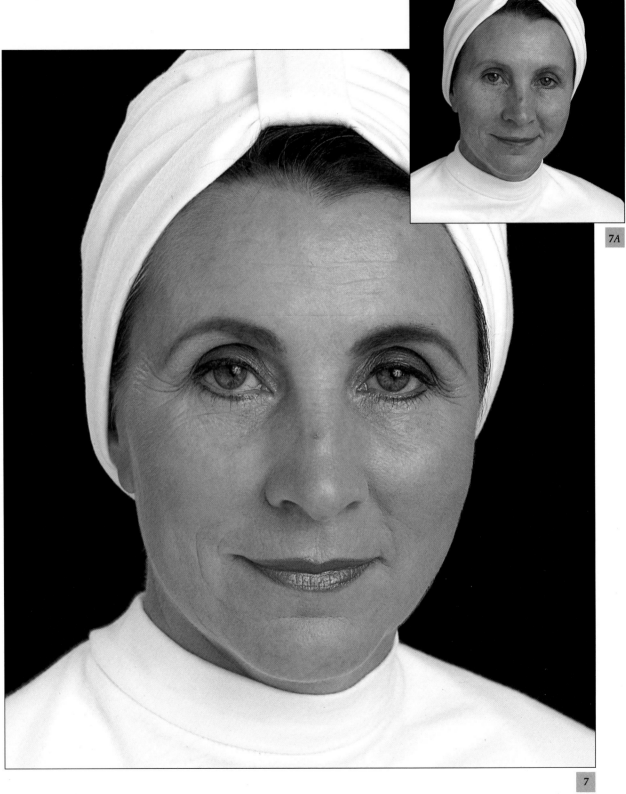

22

7A

7

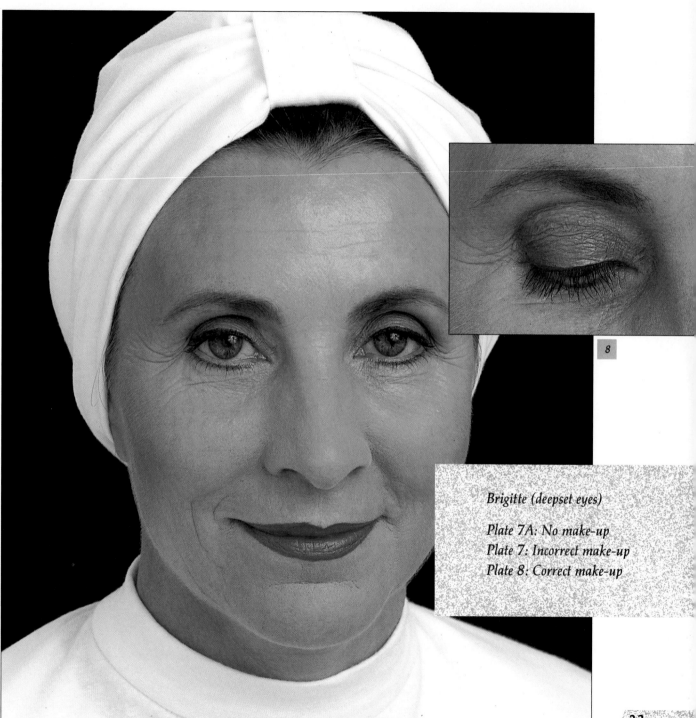

8

Brigitte (deepset eyes)

Plate 7A: No make-up
Plate 7: Incorrect make-up
Plate 8: Correct make-up

23

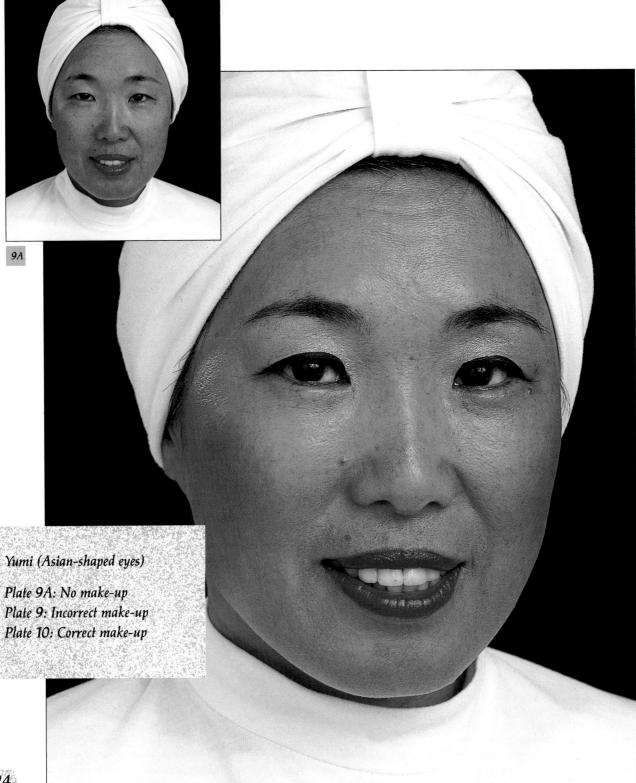

Yumi (Asian-shaped eyes)

Plate 9A: No make-up
Plate 9: Incorrect make-up
Plate 10: Correct make-up

24

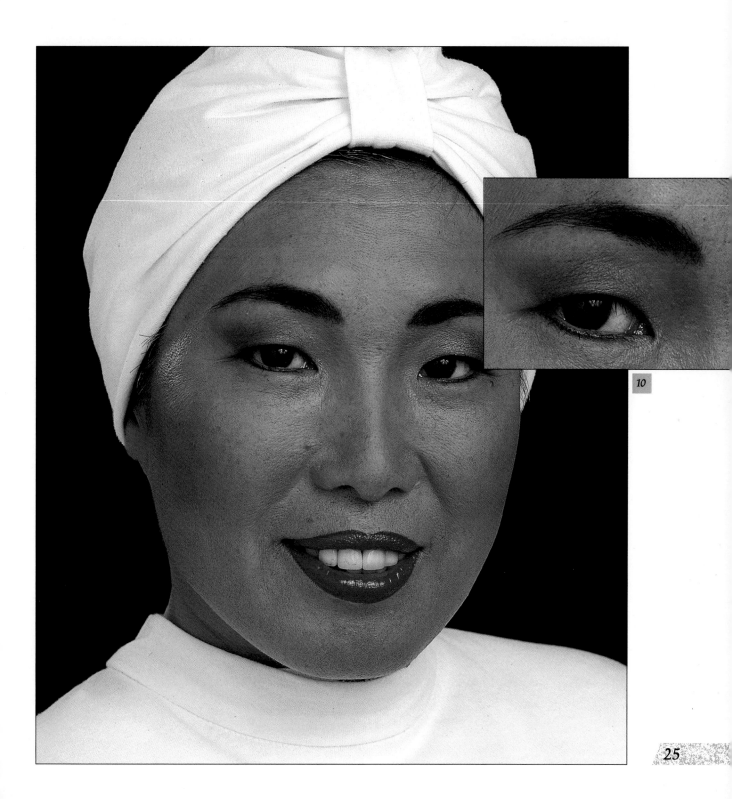

10

25

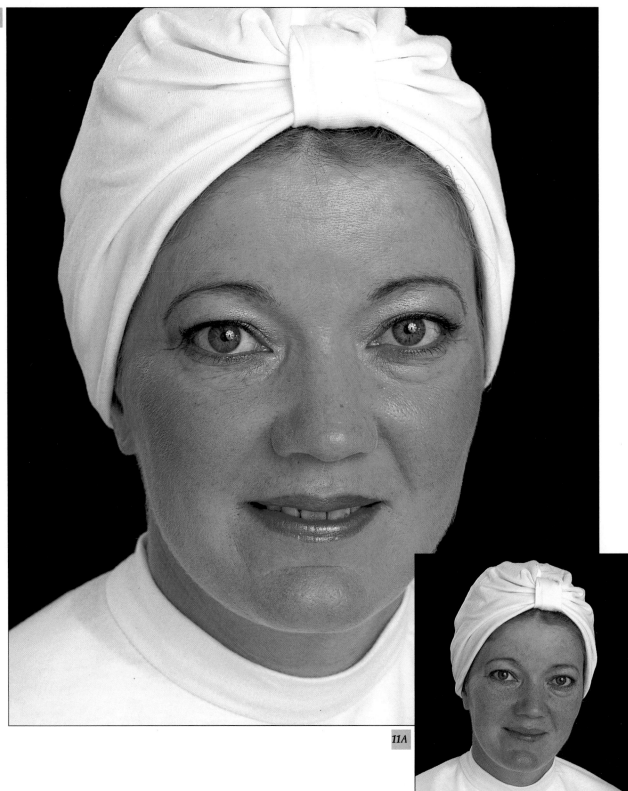

11

26

11A

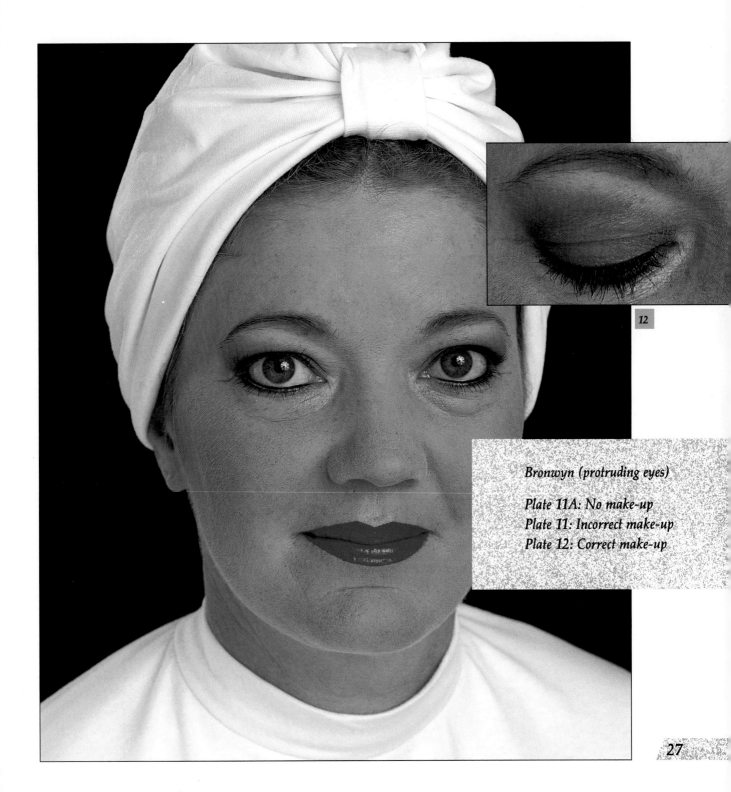

12

Bronwyn (protruding eyes)

Plate 11A: No make-up
Plate 11: Incorrect make-up
Plate 12: Correct make-up

27

Eyeshadow Combination C...

Light eyeshadows

	L1	L2	L3	L4	L5
D1	YES	YES	NO	YES	⭐ YES
D2	YES	YES	NO	YES	YES
D3	YES	YES	YES	YES	NO
D4	NO	YES	NO	NO	YES
D5	YES	YES	NO	NO	NO
D6	YES	YES	YES	YES	YES
D7	YES	YES	⭐ YES	YES	⭐ YES

Deep eyeshadows

rt

© NOUK TAYLER-VIEIRA 1991

L6	L7	L8	L9
YES	YES	YES	YES
YES	YES	YES	YES
NO	YES	YES	YES
YES	YES	YES	YES
NO	NO	NO	YES
YES	YES	YES	▪ YES
YES	YES	YES	YES

K E Y

YES — *Recommended combination*
NO — *Not a recommended combination*
✪ — *Recommended for dark skin*
▪ — *Especially recommended for women over 45 years*

NOTE: *These are suggestions only. Please feel free to select as you wish.*

Eyeliner Colour Combinatior

Most suitable eyeshadow combinations	BLUE		BLUE/GREEN	
	Upper lid	Lower lid	Upper lid	Lower lid
L1 & D3/D5	EL1	or EL3 / D1	EL1	EL2
L1 & D6/D7	EL1	D6	EL1	D6
L2 & D2/D4	EL1	or D1 / EL3	EL1	D1
L3 & D6/D7 *Evening combination	EL1	or EL3 / D6	EL1	or EL2 / D6
L4 & D1/D2/D3	or EL1 / D1	or EL3 / D1	or EL1 / D1	D1
L4 & D6/D7	EL1	D6	EL1	D6
L5 & D1/D2	or EL1 / D1	or EL3 / D1	or EL1 / D1	D1
L5 & D6/D7	EL1	D6	EL1	D6
L6 & D1/D2	or EL1 / D1	or D1 / EL3	or EL / D1	D1
L6 & D6/D7	EL1	D6	EL	D6
L7 & D1/D2	or EL1 / D1	or D1 / EL3	or EL1 / D1	D1
L7 & D6/D7	EL1	D6	EL1	D6
L8 & D6/D7 *Evening combination	EL1	or D6 / EL3	EL1	or D6 / EL2
L9 & D1, 2, 3, 4, 5	or EL1 / D1	or EL3 / D1	or EL1 / D1	D1
L9 & D6/D7 *Women over 45	EL1	D6	EL1	D6

Chart

EYE COLOURS

GREEN		BROWN	
Upper lid	**Lower lid**	**Upper lid**	**Lower lid**
or EL1 / D1	D1	or EL1 / D1	D1
EL1	D6	EL1	D6
EL1	D1	EL1	D1
EL1	D6	EL1	D6
EL1	D1	EL1	D1
EL1	D6	EL1	D6
EL1	D1	EL1	D1
EL1	D6	EL1	D6
or EL1 / D1	D1	or EL1 / D1	D1
EL1	D6	EL1	D6
or EL1 / D1	D1	or EL1 / D1	D1
EL1	D6	EL1	D6
EL1	D6	EL1	D6
or EL1 / D1	D1	or EL1 / D1	D1
EL1	D6	EL1	D6

1 Select your two best 'eyeshadow combinations' from the eyeshadow (natural compatible) colour chart.

2 Select your best eyeliner colour (either upper liner or lower liner) by first finding which group your eye colour belongs, ie, blue, blue/green, green or brown.

3 In the left hand column find your selected eyeshadow combination, ie,
a) I have blue eyes
b) my selected eyeshadows are L1 & D3.

4 Look across your eyeliner chart to find which best eyeliner colours correspond to your eyeshadow and eye colour, ie, my best eyeliner colours would be EL1 on top lid, EL3 or D1 on the lower lid.

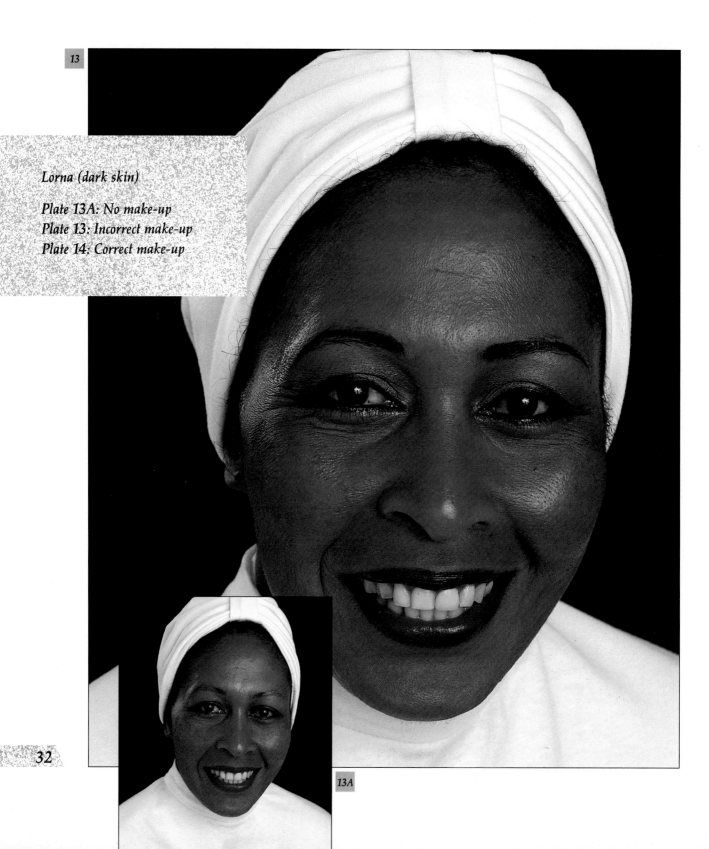

Lorna (dark skin)

Plate 13A: No make-up
Plate 13: Incorrect make-up
Plate 14: Correct make-up

13

32

13A

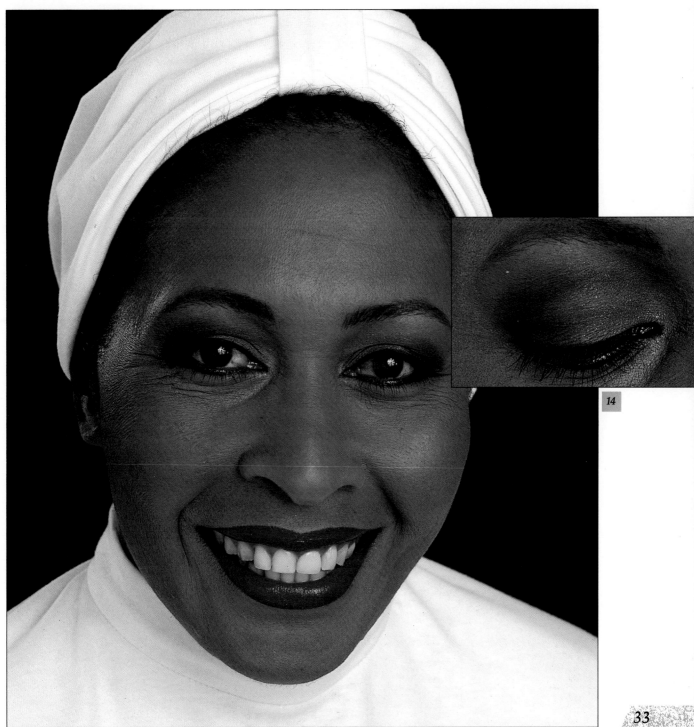

14

33

Natural Compatible Colours

lipstick colour chart

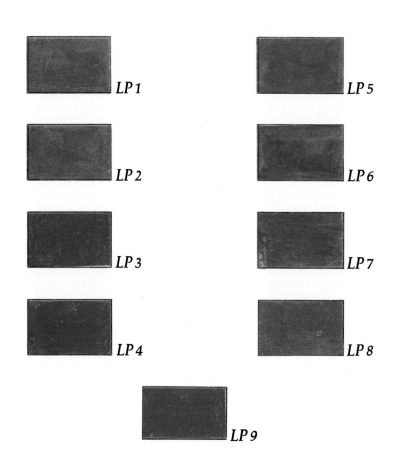

LP 1

LP 5

LP 2

LP 6

LP 3

LP 7

LP 4

LP 8

LP 9

blush colours

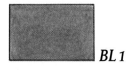

BL 1

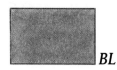

BL 2

Key to Make-up Colours

To find out the actual colours used on the models in *See How It Looks*, look at the key below and refer to the Natural Compatible Colours charts on pages 20-1 and 34.

Jan (Plate 2)

Blush	BL1		
Eyeshadows	Light: L1	Deep: D6	
Shadow liners	Upper lid: EL1	Lower lid: D6	
Lipstick	LP9		

Joanne (Plate 4)

Blush	BL1		
Eyeshadows	Light: L7	Deep: D2	
Shadow liners	Upper lid: EL1	Lower lid: EL2	
Lipstick	LP3		

Evelyne (Plate 6)

Blush	BL1		
Eyeshadows	Light: L9	Deep: D6	
Shadow liners	Upper lid: EL1	Lower lid: D6	
Lipstick	Mix of LP4 & LP9		

Brigitte (Plate 8)

Blush	BL2

Eyeshadows	Light: L4	Deep: D6
Shadow liners	Upper lid: EL1	Lower lid: EL2
Lipstick	LP5	

Yumi (Plate 10)

Blush	BL2	
Eyeshadows	Light: L1	Deep: D3
Shadow liners	Upper lid: EL1	Lower lid: D1
Lipstick	LP1	

Bronwyn (Plate 12)

Blush	BL1	
Eyeshadows	Light: L1	Deep: D2
Shadow liners	Upper lid: EL1	Lower lid: D1
Lipstick	LP2	

Lorna (Plate 14)

Blush	BL1	
Eyeshadows	Light: L8	Deep: D7
Shadow liners	Upper lid: EL1	Lower lid: EL1
Lipstick	LP4	

Colour

colour and fashion (the big con)

*I*f a brilliant blue foundation base came into fashion, would you wear it? Ask yourself these questions:

▰ Would this brilliant blue foundation base enhance your best features?

▰ Would it give you a more youthful appearance?

▰ Would it help you look more naturally beautiful?

▰ Would it give you a healthier and more vital look?

The answer to all of these questions is 'No'; it certainly would do none of these things!

You're probably astonished at the absolute stupidity of the above question, perhaps thinking, "Who'd be so gullible as to purchase, let alone wear, a brilliant blue foundation base?" And if you think that the idea of a huge make-up market for a brilliant blue foundation base is positively ludicrous, then, I've got news for you!

The brilliant blue that has been the best-seller for decades in the enormous eyeshadow market does for your eyes exactly what a brilliant blue foundation base would do for your face. All greens, aquas and silver/greys also do for your eyes what brilliant blue foundation would do for your skin.

So, if you're one of the millions of women, world-wide, who've been brainwashed into thinking these particular eyeshadows will enhance your true beauty, then it's about time you were given the cold, hard facts about the Ageing Colours.

Ageing colours: the bestsellers

We have all looked closely at a portrait painting and marvelled at how the artist managed to capture that individual on canvas, particularly if it's a young, vibrant individual, or an older person whose face is etched with character and age.

You can be sure that the clever use of colour plays a major role in the realism of such portraits. When painting an aged person, the artist would probably have incorporated shades of blue, green or grey into the shadow areas of the face. Dark or heavy shading would also have been used in certain areas to achieve an aged or tired appearance.

These same principles of colour and shading apply to make-up application. If you wear blue, green or silver/grey eyeshadow, you will look older and more tired. For the ageing eyeshadows to avoid, see the Decorative Eye-shadow Colours, pages 14-15.

If you apply a foundation base that is darker than your natural skin tone, you also stand a high chance of:

- ◢ looking older and more tired; and

- ◢ making any skin imperfection you have, such as lines, wrinkles or blotches, appear more prominent.

Frosted purple, pale, pale pink or pale, pale orange lipsticks are also wonderful for adding a decade or two to your age. Yet you'll find these colours in nearly every range of make-up. And they sell well, too!

> NOTE: *If you're under 25, you may be able to wear 'ageing colours' and still look alright. It's possible for you to wear successfully many of the colours I don't recommend. However, you will achieve a more natural and healthy looking make-up by following the guidelines in this book.*

Now you know the colours to avoid, you need to find out what other colours there are, and how to select the ones most suitable for you.

Are you cool, warm or confused?

Another area of uncertainty in make-up colour selection has been the 'cool and warm' colour theory. For over 10 years, all my make-up tuitions and seminars were backed by a sound knowledge of the 'cool and warm' colour theory. For those of you not familiar with it, here's a brief explanation.

Put in its simplest terms, for all skin colours, there are two skin undertone categories: those that have a cool undertone (blue) and those with a warm undertone (yellow).

Those with a cool undertone are better served by certain 'cooler' shades of clothing such as cool blues, pinks, silvers and greys. Those with a warm undertone look better in 'warmer' tones such as golds, apricots, yellows, greens and rusts.

It's a great theory, and has long been believed to be accurate, with 'suitable' colour

> NOTE: *For more information on best colours, see Eyes: The best colours, page 50. Eyeliners are eye definers and are not in the same colour category as eye-shadows. See Eyelining page 60.*

categories stereotyped in areas such as wardrobe, hair colour and, to a certain degree, make-up.

I say accurate for make-up to only 'a certain degree', because I have made a great discovery which gradually came about, only after experimentation with the help of thousands of women over a period of 10 years.

I have discovered that colour coding (using the warm/cool theory) does not necessarily apply to eyeshadow and foundation, whereas it works well as a guide for selecting lipstick and blush colours.

This is big news for all you faithful colour-coded converts, because you could inadvertently be ageing yourself, believing you are using the correct colours on your face.

As I asked earlier, what is the use of your make-up being totally colour co-ordinated when you risk looking tired, washed-out and older than you really are?

Turn to Plate 8, page 23 to see proof of how a 'cool' woman has been made to look five or more years younger using my technique of harmonising eye make-up with her eye colour and not her clothing. Refer to the Eyeshadow Combination Chart on pages 28-9 for your best colour selections and combinations.

NOTE: *For more information on colour selection in foundation, blush and lipstick, see the following: Foundation pages 72-5, and Powder, page 76; Blush, pages 78-9; and Lipstick, pages 86-7.*

Balance

what's balance got to do with make-up?

Have you ever seen a woman with a tiny little mouth and huge, wide eyes, over-exaggerated with lengthened shadow or eyeliner? I have!

Most of us are a mixed bag of features. This is as it should be; otherwise so-called beauty would become monotonous and boring. But to focus on these features to the best advantage, we need to look at their balance.

Mistakes with make-up are often made when certain features are overemphasised. In my example, the woman knew she had beautiful, large eyes, but fell into the trap of overplaying them, which in turn underplayed her small mouth. She created the illusion that her mouth was even smaller than it was.

Eyebrows are another feature where balance is important. A little attention to detail can make a special feature out of something quite ordinary, even without using make-up. (See Eyebrows, pages 69-71.)

As you read through and practise the information in this book, you will become an expert at applying the rules of balance to your make-up.

NOTE: *To find out how to balance eyes with lips, see The Balancing Act — eyes and lips, page 83.*

Light & Shade
focus on your features

Shading involves applying a deeper colour to an area in order to diminish it. Highlighting is the opposite; a lighter shade is used to bring the area forward.

THE MYTH OF THE SEVEN BASIC FACE SHAPES

In nearly all the make-up books and fashion magazines, the subject of face shapes and how to change them is one of the first on the list. The myth goes like this:

In the following diagram (Fig 1), there are seven basic face shapes, and the darker areas indicate where shading (or diminishing) is considered desirable to achieve the so-called 'perfect' face shape … oval.

The oval face shape has long been held to be the most desirable and therefore, to achieve this 'perfect' look, you must shape and shade your face accordingly. Well, I don't know about you, but I think the world would be a pretty boring and unattractive place if all women had an oval face. The big news is that I can help you look more attractive, whatever your face shape; and you don't need shading or highlighting to achieve it.

Interested? The next diagram (Fig 2) reveals that there are only two face shapes that should concern you; and this is only of use in discovering how to apply your blush. (See Blush — enhance your natural skin tone, page 80.)

"But what do I do if I have a round or triangular face shape?", you may ask. "How do I look attractive without light and shade?"

Over the past 10 years I have discovered a new practical theory and method which I call 'feature-focusing' and 'flaw detracting'.

Feature-focusing and flaw-detracting

The object of this method is to draw attention away from any aspects of your face that you consider to be flaws; for example, wrinkles,

OPPOSITE: **Fig 1. The old 'myth' of the seven basic face shapes.**

OVERPAGE: **In the 'two face shapes theory' there are only two facial dimensions with which the everyday woman need be concerned. The narrow and broad shapes make it easy to determine the length of your blush.**

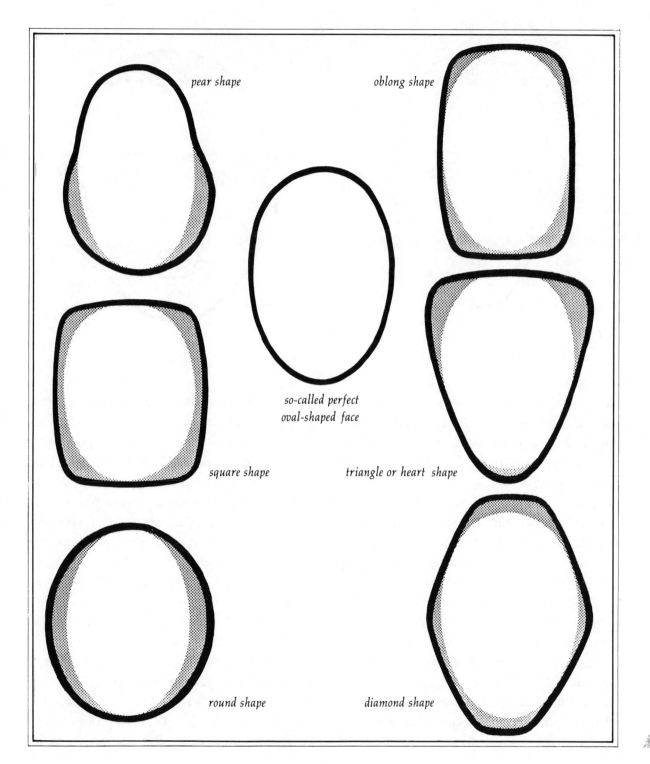

pear shape

oblong shape

so-called perfect
oval-shaped face

square shape

triangle or heart shape

round shape

diamond shape

41

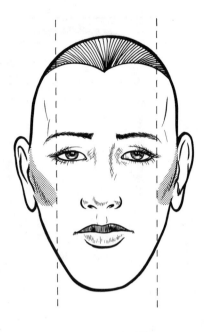

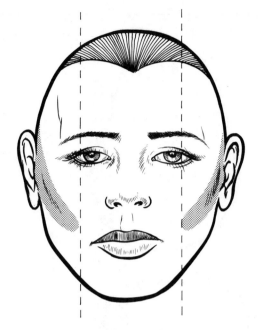

NARROW FACE   BROAD FACE

lines, a large face, a thin face, a prominent nose, or blemishes. I call this flaw-detracting. You achieve this by using the technique of feature-focusing; that is, playing up your positive features.

It's a great method as it allows you to concentrate on your favourite features and does not require you to apply great amounts of make-up to disguise any less desired ones.

Everyone is different, but if you want to get the best out of your individual make-up, then there are two main features on which to focus. First, your eyes; second, your mouth.

These are the two predominant areas of your face to which other people are attracted almost immediately. The eyes hold a special attraction because we communicate with them virtually all the time. With feature-focusing,

you'll learn how to focus masterfully on these features, eliminating the focus on wrinkles, lines, blemishes, face shapes and prominent noses. These so-called flaws will seem to fade into the background. It's a more natural, and individual way of enhancing your best points.

For a photographic example of how the theory of feature-focusing and flaw-detraction works, see Joanne in Plate 3, page 16. Joanne has a round face. Look at Plate 4. Without using shading to change her face shape, I concentrated on her other features and, as you can see for yourself, her face looks thinner.

If you're concerned about shading and highlighting of your nose or chin, let's look at another example. Study Jan in Plate 1. Jan was always searching for new products and techniques to disguise the size of her nose.

Look at her with incorrect make-up. Notice her nose? Now, in Plate 2, see her with a feature-focusing make-up. What takes your attention? Her beautiful eyes! You don't even look at her nose, do you?

Jan knows now that altering the appearance of her nose shape by shading and highlighting is out of the question.

For those who are still not convinced about throwing away your shading and highlighting tricks, let me explain an important point. Facial shading and highlighting is frequently used in the world of photography, television, films and the theatre. It works well in these media, with the added tricks of soft-focus lenses and diffused lighting helping to soften edges and make the face appear more 'natural'. Conversely, in everyday life, if you use heavy corrective make-up techniques of highlight and shade to change the shape of your face and features, then you will look hard, unnatural and probably theatrical.

Now you have the licence you were looking for to appreciate yourself as you are, with no reason to feel less attractive because you have the 'wrong' face shape or a pronounced nose or chin.

Put my theories and the methods in this book into practice, along with your positive affirmations, and you will be well on the way to looking uniquely beautiful.

Eyes need light and shade

An important focus area of light and shade is eye make-up. This is the one area of the face where the use of light and shade could make or break your total make-up. Incorrect eye make-up application can result in the illusion that 'The lights are on but nobody's home'.

Eyes

your most important feature

Which one facial feature can communicate so many of your emotions — joy, sadness, anger, surprise, hatred and love? Which one facial feature can frown, wink, cry and laugh? Which one feature can be the window to your soul, communicating the very best that is you? Answer: Your eyes!

Because the correct application of eye make-up is of such importance in the success of your appearance, many myths must be exploded. Knowing its importance, unlike the authors of many make-up books, I've decided to make eye make-up the introductory subject in our make-up journey. (To learn the correct 'sequence' in the application of a full make-up, you will find the answers in the latter part of this book.)

A large portion of this book is devoted to the application and selection of eye make-up because:

1   Your eyes are your most important facial feature.

2   Eye make-up has been, up until now, the most difficult area of make-up for most women.

3   Eye make-up is the area of most confusion due to poor and incorrect education available.

Let's talk about eye make-up education. Depending on the advice you have been given about colour selection and application, you will either achieve a youthful, natural look because you possess an understanding of colour selection and the correct application techniques, or you will fail miserably.

Unfortunately, make-up colour selection, and in particular eyeshadow colours, follows the whims of fashion. As I said earlier, you could well be ageing yourself and making yourself look tired or ill by purchasing unsuitable colours.

As far as application is concerned, you have probably heard nothing about light and shade and precious little about its role in creating beautiful eye make-up. On the other hand, you may have heard of and/or experimented with half a dozen outdated theories, all much the same and leaving you wondering whether it's all worthwhile.

In this chapter, you will learn the three basic principles to successful eye make-up.

EYESHADOW
What shape are your eyes in?

Of all the make-up areas, eyeshadow is by far the most challenging, enlightening and rewarding. The three major factors that govern its successful application are:

1   The use of light and shade.

2   The use of colour.

3   Easy application techniques.

Let's discuss the first. What is your eye shape? Knowing your eye shape will tell you where to apply light and deep eyeshadows. Use your mirror, and make sure you are in good, clear light — either daylight or fluorescent.

Do you have a small eyelid or a large one? Is it protruding or receding? As you see in Fig 1, the lid area extends from the eyelashes to the crease or socket, and the brow area from the socket to the eyebrow.

The objective here is to find out which area appears larger. If it is your lid, then see if it's deep-set or protruding. Does your lid area recede a little or is the brow area more prominent?

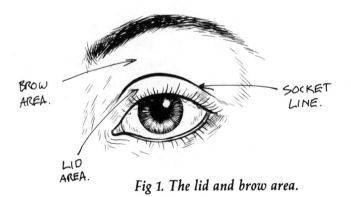

BROW AREA.

SOCKET LINE.

LID AREA.

Fig 1. The lid and brow area.

I want you to look at Fig 2 and see which eye shape is closest to yours. Select one and stay with it. We will return to your eye shape after we finish with light and shade.

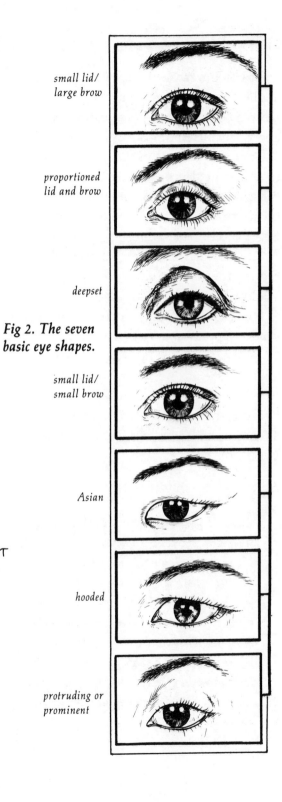

small lid/ large brow

proportioned lid and brow

deepset

Fig 2. The seven basic eye shapes.

small lid/ small brow

Asian

hooded

protruding or prominent

45

Light and deep eyeshadows

Light colours make the area to which they're applied appear larger and bring it forward. Deep colours do the opposite, making the area appear smaller and pushing it back.

Now you know this rule, where, in order to achieve balance, would you put your light eyeshadow if you had a small lid and a larger brow area? Which area would you try to make larger and bring forward?

The answer, of course, is the lid. And to reduce the brow area, you'd apply a deeper shadow in the socket area of the brow.

For examples of incorrect and correct shadow application, refer back to Plate 1, page 12. Jan has a small lid and large brow area. You can see in the incorrect photo that her eyes look tired and heavy-lidded. That's because she applied her deeper shade to her already small lid and her lighter shadow to her large brow area.

> NOTE: *If you are concerned about either close-set or wide-set eyes, forget the shading techniques you may have learned in the past. I find these techniques unsatisfactory and feel they draw attention to the very area you wish to minimise. My method of feature-focusing enhances the beauty of your eyes, and will have the effect of making the 'space flaw' between your eyes appear to fade away. Try it!*

Now look at the correct make-up in Plate 2, page 13. What a difference! You can see what it's done for Jan's eyes. They're open, bright and balanced. The lighter colour was applied to her lid and the deeper shade to the socket area of her brow.

Master eye diagrams for eyeshadow application

To make it easier for you to find out where to apply the light and deep eyeshadows, I've divided the usual seven eye shapes into two groups (which is probably totally different

> NOTE: *If you're under 25, with a medium-size lid and brow area, that neither recedes nor protrudes (a proportioned lid and brow), then you can successfully use methods of light and shade application for Group 1 and Group 2.*

from anything you've ever read before). If you have a smaller lid area than brow area, or deep-set eyes, then you'll belong to Group 1. Refer to the Two Master Eye Diagrams on page 47.

If you have a fairly large eyelid that is more prominent or protruding, then you'll belong to Group 2.

Blush shadows

As I said earlier, we tend to have shadowy areas around the eyes which intensify as we get older. To use blue, green and grey eyeshadows

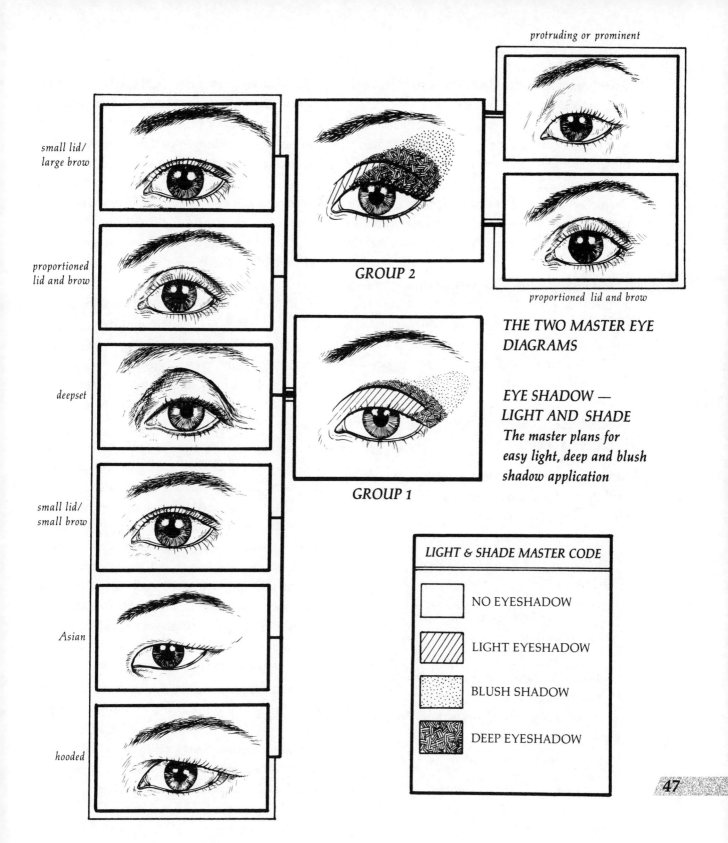

small lid/
large brow

proportioned
lid and brow

deepset

small lid/
small brow

Asian

hooded

protruding or prominent

GROUP 2

proportioned lid and brow

**THE TWO MASTER EYE
DIAGRAMS**

**EYE SHADOW —
LIGHT AND SHADE**
*The master plans for
easy light, deep and blush
shadow application*

GROUP 1

LIGHT & SHADE MASTER CODE

NO EYESHADOW

LIGHT EYESHADOW

BLUSH SHADOW

DEEP EYESHADOW

47

only increases the problem (refer to the Ageing Colours, Plate 3, page 13).

To add a touch of warmth and magnetism to the eyes, I always apply blush. Even by itself, blush on the eyes is a great lift, softly and subtly brushed on the upper, outer corners of the brow area. For your convenience, I have included one of these blush shadows in the colour chart. I designed this colour specifically for use on the eye.

You'll notice that for both groups, applying a touch of blush to the upper, outer corner of the brow area (see Lid and Brow diagram, Fig 1, page 45) is recommended. (See the Natural Compatible Colours chart, pages 20-1, for the blush shadow colour.)

Eyeshadows: the terrible frosts, the beautiful matts

Now you've got the idea of where your light and deep eyeshadows go, we'll look at the effects of light and shade.

NOTE: *No highlighter or light colour is applied directly under the eyebrow. The brow already protrudes slightly; adding highlight would make this area appear larger and more prominent. This would detract from the natural beauty of the eye.*

You know now that light makes an area appear larger and brings the area forward. Did you know, however, that frosted (shiny, iridescent) eyeshadows add light, reflect light, and make the frosted area come forward and appear larger? Well, they do! Unfortunately, approximately 80 per cent of eyeshadows are frosted, which creates a bit of a problem for you if you're looking for a deep shadow colour with which to shade your eyes.

There are no frosted, deeper colours which will help to achieve the desired result of a deep shadow — that is, to make an area recede or to shade it. If you're using a frosted deep colour on your eyes, it totally defeats the purpose of putting a deep shadow there in the first place. Keep away from all frosted eyeshadows. They do nothing for you.

If you're over 25, then you may have noticed a slight crêpe-like appearance or looseness of the skin on your lid and brow area. This is normal, but the looseness and crêpiness will definitely be intensified if you apply a frosted shadow to the socket and brow area. Frosted shadow on these areas will make your eyes appear old and wrinkled, even if they're not. They are ageing and theatrical. Look at Evelyne in Plate 6 (page 18, incorrect make-up). You can see that the frosted shadow has intensified crêpiness and wrinkles on her eye area.

Before purchasing an eyeshadow, test it in daylight or fluorescent light. Using a brush, 'paint' your fingertip heavily with the desired shadow colour. Now hold your fingertip towards the light. You'll soon see if the shadow is excessively frosted — it will glitter.

What about lightly pearlised eyeshadows? These shadows have some reflective qualities but you would have to look at them in daylight to notice it.

In contrast to frosted, deep shadows, the light-coloured pearl shadows uplift the eye, whatever the wearer's age (as long as they're applied to the lid only).

- Deep colours — Choose a matt (no shine) finish, not frosted.

- Light colours — Choose a matt or light pearl (not heavily frosted) finish.

- Blush (blush shadow) for eyes — A matt finish is preferred.

If you look again at Evelyne's photos on pages 18-19, you'll see on page 19 that she looks much younger and healthier after applying matt eyeshadows rather than frosted ones.

Where do you purchase matt eyeshadows? They are scarce. But, don't despair! You will find information in this book explaining where to obtain these colours.

Share your new-found knowledge with other women and keep asking for what you want from cosmetic manufacturers. As more and more women are getting to be beautifully older and wiser, more matt shadows will emerge on the make-up market. It's about time the manufacturers gave us what we want.

The useless medium-intensity eyeshadow colours

A huge proportion of the eyeshadows produced and sold fall into the category of medium-intensity colours or, as I like to call them, the 'useless' colours. They join other non-wearable eyeshadow groups such as the ageing colours and the frosteds.

Useless, medium-intensity eyeshadow colours don't create any sort of depth or life in your eye make-up. They are just pretty colours that look wonderful in the packet. Why? Because of one or other of the following:

1 They are not light enough (and cannot highlight the eye).

2 They are too light and look hard and ageing.

3 They are not deep enough, and, therefore, cannot shade the eye.

So, don't be fooled by these seductive colours. All they will give your eyes is a 'flat' appearance. To illustrate my point, look at Bronwyn's eye make-up in Plate 11 (page 26, incorrect make-up). The attractive duo pack of pink and mauve eyeshadows she applied is an example of the 'useless' shadow colours which do nothing to enhance natural beauty. For examples of useless eyeshadows, refer to the Decorative Eyeshadow Colours, pages 14-15.

Given that most of the eyeshadows produced world-wide, fall into one or all of the categories we've recognised as useless, you can see that looking for the ideal eyeshadows is something of a challenge.

To help you meet this challenge, I suggest that you don't buy any more duo, trio or quad eyeshadow compacts. They are nothing but a con trick. Most of these multi packs contain examples of ageing, useless or frosted products. However gorgeous they may look sitting innocently in the pack, don't be tempted. I recommend you buy only singles. That way you can select light or deep shadows, your best colours and matt shadows.

THE BEST COLOURS
Taking the fear out of change

After reading the bad news on ageing, useless and frosted eyeshadows, you're probably thinking: "Well, what eyeshadow colours are left?" and, "Whatever colours they are, I certainly haven't seen them around much."

You probably haven't seen them because most eyeshadows on the market until now have been the colours that I don't recommend. As you'll see in the Decorative Eyeshadow Colour Chart (pages 14-15), the majority of eyeshadows you've been attracted to probably belong to the useless, ageing or frosted category. This group of no-no eyeshadows is largely regarded as 'safe' by most women. The perception is that they're commonly available and easy to co-ordinate with your clothing.

What about the new eyeshadow colours on the Natural Compatible Colours chart (pages 20-1)? Do you feel comfortable with the thought of applying these to your eyes? If you do, then that's great. But, if you don't, let me guess why. You may feel:

1   "They're too 'dark'. I might look as if I have a black eye."

2   "They're just not the colours I would have selected for my eyes."

3   "What about colour co-ordinating with my clothing? What eyeshadows do I use if I'm wearing a blue or green outfit?"

4   "What if, in my application, I made a mistake? Everyone would notice it and I'd feel conspicuous."

5   "What if the fashion changes?"

If you can identify with any of these statements, it may comfort you to know that many of my clients have expressed to me those very same fears about the new eyeshadow colours. They, too, were sceptical at first, but what they did was try these colours once. From then on, their fears dissolved.

Relax! It's normal to feel uneasy about moving away from the eyeshadow colours with which you feel comfortable. All you have to do is decide to try the new shadows. The results will give you renewed confidence.

Here's a simple exercise to help you see the effects of the 'bad' shadow colours and the 'good' shadow colours in contrast to each other. Apply make-up to one entire half of your face using eyeshadow colours from the ageing, frosted or useless colours.

On the other side of your face, apply a full make-up using my recommended technique and eyeshadows from the new natural, compatible range. Remember where to apply the light and deep colours. Refer to the Master Eye Diagrams on page 47.

You'll see the difference immediately. Which half of your face looks more vibrant, attractive and, perhaps, younger? For more examples of this eyeshadow colour technique, see:

Jan (small lid/large brow), Plate 2, page 13

Joanne (small lid/small brow), Plate 4, page 17

Evelyne (mature, small lid/large brow), Plate 6, page 19

Brigitte (deep-set eyes), Plate 8, page 23

Yumi (Asian-shaped eyes), Plate 10, page 25

Bronwyn (protruding or prominent eyes), Plate 12, page 27

Lorna (dark skin, small lid/large brow), Plate 14, page 33

Accompanying these correct make-up photos are photos of the incorrect application. Please study the differences between the two.

Eyeshadow colour: recommended combinations

Perhaps you've looked at the natural, compatible eyeshadow colours and thought they were great, but puzzled over how to select the best combinations for your eyes.

There's no need to worry about this as I have prepared a separate Eyeshadow Combination Chart to help you simply and quickly select eyeshadow combinations that work for you. You'll find the chart on pages 28-9.

Your eye colour

The good news about the natural, compatible colours is that they harmonise with all eye colours, be they green, blue, black, brown or a combination of these.

You might be asking now, "What about co-ordinating my eye make-up with my clothing?

Are there colours in the new shadow range that will match?" If your outfit is green or blue, then the answer is a flat 'no'.

Matching eyeshadow with the colour of your outfit is a total waste of time and not beauty enhancing (unless, by chance, you're wearing an outfit that's the same colour as your best shadow colour).

How to select your colours

If you want to enhance the natural beauty of your eyes and add a magnetic attractiveness to them with eyeshadow, then choose shadows that harmonise with your eye colour.

Eyes are either blue, green, black or brown, or a mixture of these; it is eye colour and not clothing colour that indicates your best eyeshadow colours.

You see, you don't have to match your eyeshadow with your outfit, because your eyes are magnetic on their own. They simply need

NOTE: *If you have blue/green (teal) eyes similar to those of our models, Joanne (Plate 4, page 17) and Brigitte (Plate 8, page 23), you can intensify your eye colour considerably by applying the teal-coloured shadow-liner. See Eyeliner Colour Combination Chart, colour EL2, pages 30-1. If you apply this colour along your lower lashes, it will add life and sparkle to your eye make-up. It also looks natural.*

to be made-up to enhance that effect. If you have beautifully made-up eyes and you have tried to enhance their actual colour, then it is your eyes that become your 'special feature', not your eyeshadow.

Do you ever look to see if a woman has green eyeshadow on to match her green dress? If you do happen to notice someone and she's beautifully colour co-ordinated, did you notice the colour of her eyes? You didn't, did you, because her eyeshadow colour overwhelmed that of her eyes.

Next time you're out in a crowd, look for a woman wearing either blue, green, aqua or silver eyeshadow and see which takes your attention first; her eyes, or her eyeshadow!

Eyeshadow: cream or powder?

Cream eyeshadows and pencil eyeshadows have been around for decades. There are some great colours, but when it comes to application and durability, they don't wear as well as powder shadows. Whatever your age, I recommend the use of powder eyeshadows. They are applied easily, stay on well and tend to look more natural.

Eyeshadow applications: the 'wet' and 'dry' technique

Now that we've covered which colours to select and how to combine them, it's time to explore the best way to apply them. Let's take a look at the tools available for the job.

Most commonly available are the sponge or velour applicators which are usually included in your eyeshadow compacts when you purchase them. I don't recommend them for applying eyeshadow for these reasons:

1   They tend to pull at the delicate skin of your eyelid.

2   They pick up and deposit so much colour at once that they make a soft, blended-look eye make-up almost impossible to achieve.

If you're serious about your eye make-up, I recommend the sole use of an eyeshadow brush for applying shadow. You can regulate exactly how much colour you apply and blending is made much easier. On page 53, is a diagram of the recommended eyeshadow brushes. Make sure you check the size and shape of the brush head before purchasing. A brush that's stiff, too thick or cut bluntly

NOTE: *One exception to contrasting shadow with clothing colours is never to wear an orange eyeshadow with pink clothing, and vice versa.*

NOTE: *To those of you who are over 50, be careful when using deep browns as they can be too heavy. Violets are the best deep colours and peach or peach-pinks are the best light ones.*

square at the end will only result in frustration for you.

Crease-proofing your eyeshadow

Have you ever had the following experience? It's 4 pm, you've had a busy day, you decide to freshen up quickly. But on closer inspection of your eyeshadow you realise that it hasn't yet disappeared totally, but instead deposited itself in neat little creases in the socket area of your eyes.

If this has happened to you, let me share another of my discoveries. I call it the 'wet and dry' eyeshadow application technique, and it helps eliminate eyeshadow creasing.

I discovered this technique during my film and TV make-up career. They say that necessity is the mother of invention, so, set the task of finding a solution to the creasing problem, I experimented with wetting eyeshadow before applying it — and it worked! That was eight years and over 4000 make-ups ago.

To be more specific, the only area of your eye to which you'd apply a wet or dampened shadow colour would be the eyelid, not the socket or brow. You see, the eyelid moves continually as we blink. It tends to roll back into the socket line, causing shadow to crease. So the lid is the only area to which you need to apply dampened shadow. Other advantages of the wet shadow technique are:

1   It eliminates flecks of shadow falling onto your cheeks.

2   It helps to make your eyeshadow water-resistant.

NOTE: *Before applying any eyeshadow, refer to the Master Eye Diagrams for directions on where to apply your light and deep shadows. See chart on page 47.*

For easy instructions on the wet and dry eyeshadow technique, see the steps and illustrations on the following pages, pages 54-9.

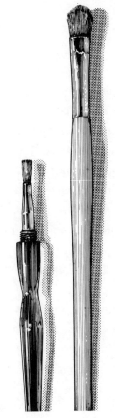

Recommended eyeshadow brushes.

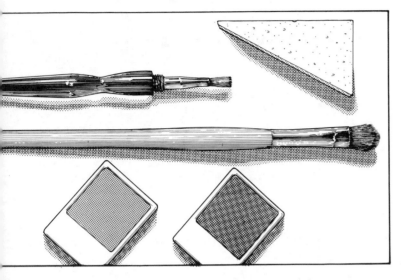

1 Tools: These are the two eyeshadow brushes I recommend and a latex wedge sponge. The sponge is used to blend your eyeshadow. The smaller of the two brushes is the size of a lip brush. This is the brush to apply 'light' colour only. (The eye-lid is the only area recommended to take 'light' colour.) The larger, tapered brush is for 'deep' shadow only.

2 Before eyeshadow, always apply foundation base and powder. If you skip this step, your shadow will be uneven in areas and quickly disappear. I suggest a panstick foundation under eye make-up. It forms a wonderful base for shadows to glide and blend on to and it helps to keep your eye make-up looking fresh and even all day long, without the need to touch-up. For those of you who never wear a foundation base on your face, but do wear eyeshadow, I still suggest you apply a base under your eye make-up.

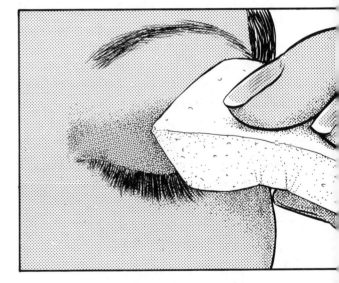

3 Using your selected 'light' colour shadow, scrape a little powder up at the corner of the compact with the end of your brush handle.

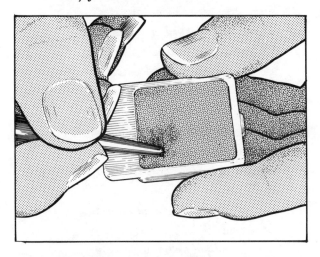

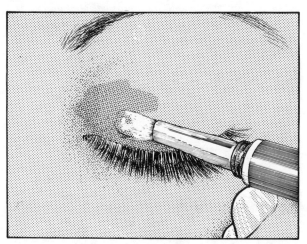

5 Now stroke shadow onto your lid area. Only apply on the area marked 'light' in your Master Eye Diagram.

6 Using your fingertip, briskly and firmly 'pat' the wet shadow, until it's well blended. If you make a mistake, simply wet your fingertip and run over the shadow to even it out.

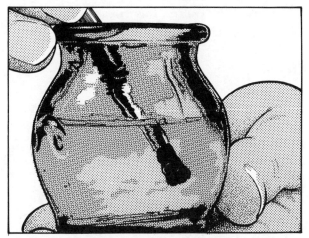

4 Take your small shadow brush (for light colour) and dip it into clean water, then squeeze out excess. Coat the damp brush well with the light shadow.

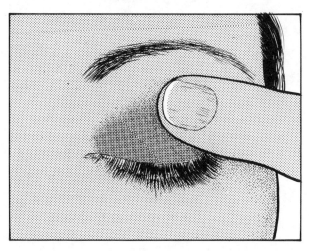

7 Apply a second coat of shadow for durability. Repeat steps 4 and 5.

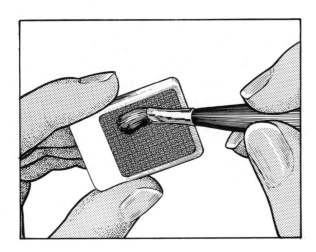

8 This is the deep shadow and is always to be applied 'dry', not wet. Using the deep shadow brush (dry) stroke into deep eyeshadow colour. Remove excess shadow from the brush, by brushing it first onto the back of the hand. (This eliminates spills on cheeks and helps you regulate how much deep colour to apply.)

Deep shadow can only be applied successfully if done in stages. Be patient and put only a little on at a time. With practice, this technique becomes fast and easy.

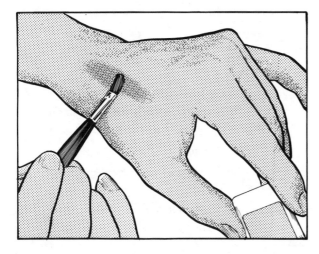

9 Begin applying your deep colour to the outer corner of your lid. Brush it inwards from the outer corner so as you don't get an 'overhang'. See Some common mistakes, pages 59-60.

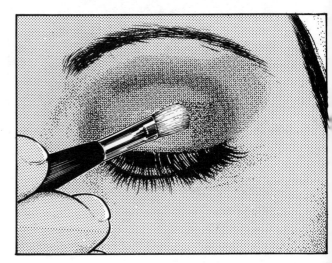

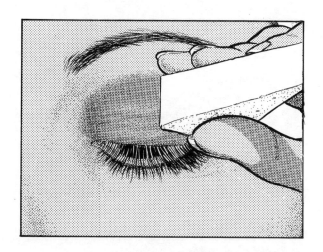

10 With the stiffest corner of your sponge, 'press and roll' gently but firmly to assist in quickly blending your deep shadow. (Don't 'pull' the skin, only 'press').

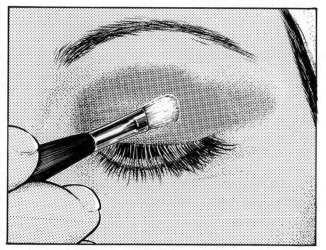

11 Add a little more deep colour to brush, dust off excess again and begin to apply colour to the socket line of the eye. Begin from the outer corner of the eye, brushing in towards the centre. (Don't take deep colour to the inner corner of the eye.)

NOTE: *If you have crepey or loose skin on your lid and socket area (or folds of skin), make sure you gently 'lift' the eye area with your fingers first before applying deep shadow. This way, you will see the socket line for easy application.*

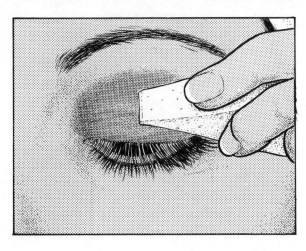

12 Blend well with sponge.

13 Repeat steps 11 and 12 to reach desired depth of colour.

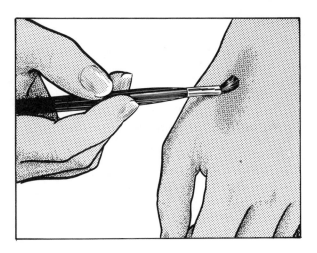

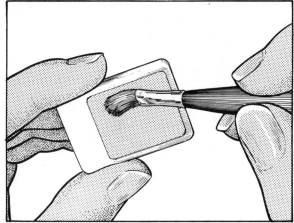

14 Once you have blended your deep shadow, dust off all deep colour onto the back of your hand. Make sure none of the deep colour is left on your brush.

15 Apply blush shadow to your dry brush; not too much, only a light coat.

16 Now apply a little blush shadow to the upper, outer corner of the eye, 'overlapping' your deep

colour in this area. Take it upwards and out, almost to the end of the brow.

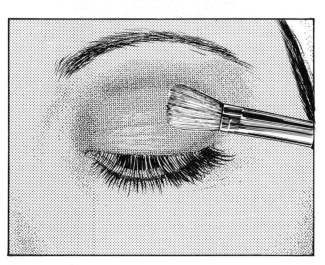

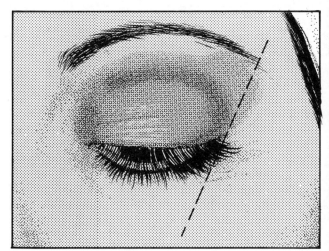

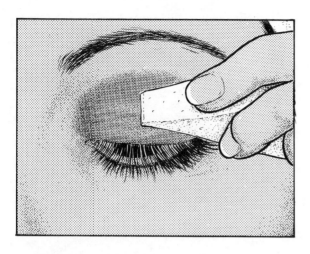

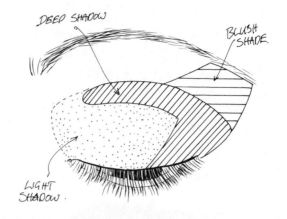

17 *Pat this area again, well, with your sponge. Make sure there are no 'hard edges'.*

Some common mistakes

1 *Applying eyeshadow on the innermost corner of the eye. This accentuates 'crêpiness', wrinkles and dark circles.*

18 *And here (with a little mascara and shadow liner) is the finished effect.*

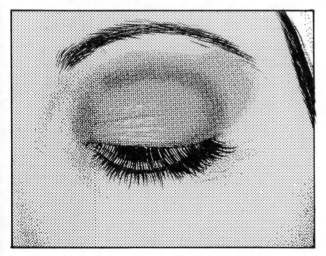

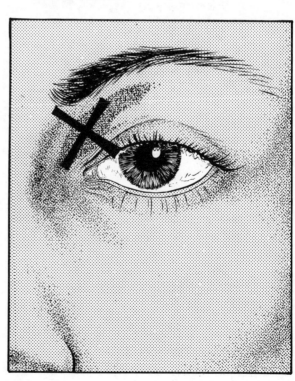

59

2 *Applying a light-coloured highlighter under the brow, which will accentuate the brow area, giving a 'protruding brow' look.*

3 *Applying eyeshadow too far past the outer corner of the eye, which will create a 'drooping effect'.*

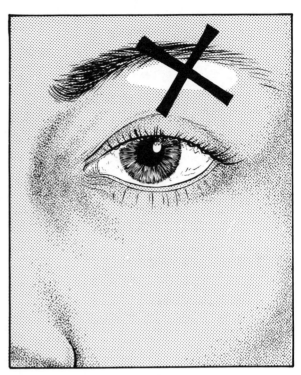

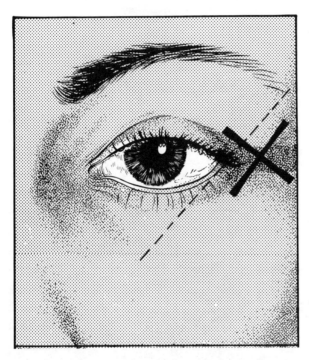

A problem most women have when applying eyeshadow is uneven distribution of colour or the appearance of colour sticking or blotching. Check the following two areas if this is a problem.

- Remove all fine brow hairs under eyebrow.
- Make sure you use a good coverage foundation base and powder under your eyeshadow.

EYELINING MADE EASY (THROW AWAY YOUR EYE-LINING PENCILS!)

Shadow-lining

Up until now, if you wanted to line your eyes, the product you'd be most likely to use would be an eye pencil.

I believe eye pencils to be one of the most difficult make-up products to use for these reasons:

- They need to be sharpened continually and they break often.
- They pull and sometimes scratch the delicate area around the eye.
- They smudge in warm weather and tend to run as the day unfolds.

- It's practically impossible to get a delicate, even line on your upper eye lid.

- They are often expensive.

Have you, too, had problems with eye pencils? If you have, the following guideline will be a welcome relief for you. Throw away your eyelining pencil and use your eyeshadows instead! Eyeshadows are absolutely wonderful for eyelining.

- They don't run like pencil.

- You don't have to sharpen them.

- They are less expensive.

- They are much more simple to apply — you don't really need a steady hand.

- They provide a softer, more muted eyeline.

- The liner lasts all day.

- Their application is gentler on the delicate eye area and doesn't pull the skin.

If you want to have that muted eyeliner look then eyeshadows are great. Also, to achieve a fine line on your upper lid you can use this method. The secret to achieving a perfect eyeliner look is to use only a professional artist's brush such as Roymac 3550 no. 3 (about $6 Australian). Don't use the common cosmetic eyeliner brushes as they splay. (See diagram of correct eyelining brush.)

Shadow-line application steps

I find this technique not only better than using pencils but also less expensive and more natural than using liner pens or liquid eyeliners.

It's a wonderful method of eyelining, especially if you wear glasses and find it difficult to see, or if you have a less than steady hand. You really can't make a mistake, as the liner is always muted and soft-looking anyway.

The liner is applied after the eyeshadow.

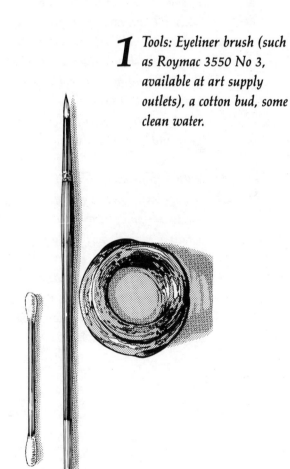

1 Tools: Eyeliner brush (such as Roymac 3550 No 3, available at art supply outlets), a cotton bud, some clean water.

Lower lid: I believe every woman will benefit from applying a little liner to their lower lid. No eye make-up is complete without this step. It is a vital step, especially for all women over 25.

2 *After selecting your shadow-liner colour, with the handle end of your brush scrape and loosen a little eyeshadow. Dampen your brush in clean water and dip it into your eyeshadow. For easy application of lower-lid line, hold your mirror up higher and look 'up' into the mirror. Now apply shadow-liner to lower lid ('under' eyelashes, not inside eye). Only line two thirds or three quarters of your lower lid; never take liner into inner corner of your eye.*

3 *With a clean dampened cotton bud, smudge lower lid line gently backwards and forwards until you obtain a 'muted', 'soft' eyelining effect. For durability, repeat application and smudge again. For a natural-look eyeliner, it is not necessary for you to line the top lid, only the bottom (smudge always).*

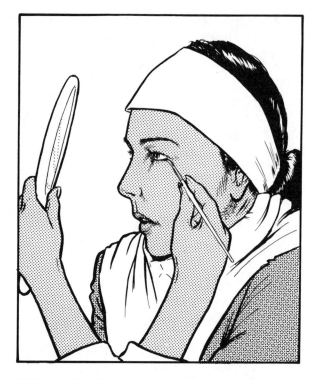

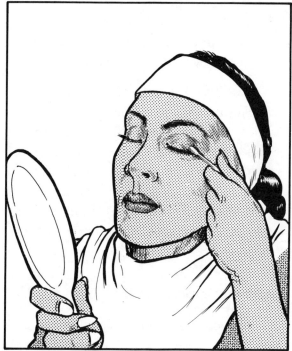

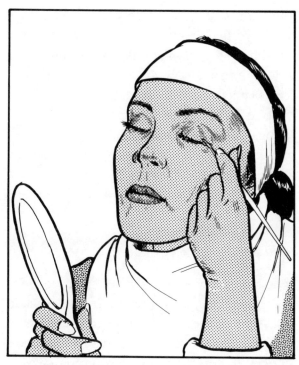

Upper eye-lid: Lining your upper eyelid is optional, but is usually advisable for evening make-up.

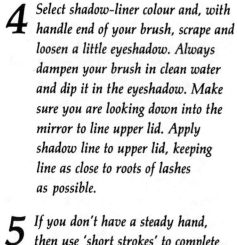

4 Select shadow-liner colour and, with handle end of your brush, scrape and loosen a little eyeshadow. Always dampen your brush in clean water and dip it in the eyeshadow. Make sure you are looking down into the mirror to line upper lid. Apply shadow line to upper lid, keeping line as close to roots of lashes as possible.

5 If you don't have a steady hand, then use 'short strokes' to complete your line, then smudge with a damp cotton bud if a smoky or smudged line is preferred. This eliminates the need for you to close one eye (this puckers the skin and breaks up your liner).

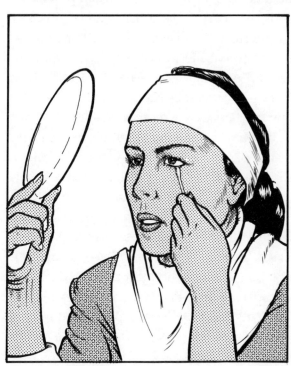

Eyeliner

The main function of eyeliner is to outline or define your eyes. If selected and applied correctly, eyeliner can enlarge, balance and define your eyes.

I recommend eyeliner for all women, even just a little under the lower lashes. Even without eyeshadow, a soft smudge of liner under the eyes can give a fresh, natural look.

Another advantage of eyeliner is that when applied to the upper lid, it can make your eyelashes appear much thicker without recourse to heavy coats of mascara.

Eyeliner colours

I wrote previously about the useless, medium-intensity eyeshadows. A huge proportion of the available eyeshadows consists of these colours and is totally useless because the tones are neither light nor deep enough to add depth and contour to your eyes. The same principle applies to eyeliner.

Because you need to give definition with an eyelining colour, you need to use a deep colour. Any light lining colour will give your eyelashes a 'bald' appearance. The useless shadow colours don't lift your eyes at all; in fact, they do the opposite. So, make sure you choose a deep shadow colour for lining. For suggested eyeliner colours, see the eyeshadow chart — the Natural Compatible Colours, page 21.

If you are still not convinced about using a deep eyelining colour to frame your eyes, try this simple test. On one eye, use a 'useless' eyelining shade (not a deep colour; perhaps a pretty blue, green or mauve). On the other eye, line in the way I've described using a deep colour eyeshadow (not frosted). Which eye looks larger and more attractive?

To assist you in selecting the best shadow-lining colours to complement your eyeshadow and eye colour, see the Eyeliner Colour Combination Chart, pages 30-1. For those of you with blue/green (teal) coloured eyes, see the Notes on page 51.

Kohl pencil

When you see 'kohl' or 'kajal' marked on a make-up pencil, it usually means that it's made to use inside the rim of the eye. However many kohl pencils can irritate sensitive eyes and are difficult to apply. Make sure when purchasing your kohl pencil that it has been ophthalmologist-tested. If you want a pencil specifically to line the inside rim of your eye, then don't use an 'eyelining' one. These are formulated to be used on the exterior of the eye — to line the outside and not the inside of the eye.

If you're wondering whether or not to use a kohl pencil, then I'll help you decide. Lining the inside of the eye can either make the eye appear small or make it appear more defined. The larger the eye, the more effective kohl will be. If you have small eyes, kohl will tend to make them look even smaller. If you're still not sure, look in the mirror directly, and see if you have a high, medium or low-set iris. (The iris is the coloured part of your eye). This is demonstrated in more detail in the illustration on page 65.

1 *High-set iris (kohl pencil can work well here).*

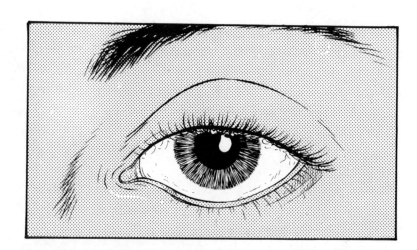

2 *Medium-set iris (kohl pencil can work if eye is large).*

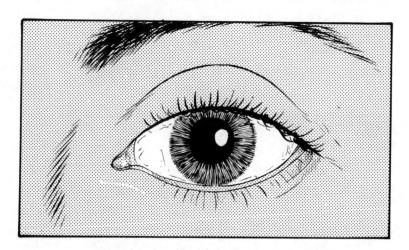

3 *Low-set iris (kohl pencil is not recommended as it will give the illusion of a closed or small eye).*

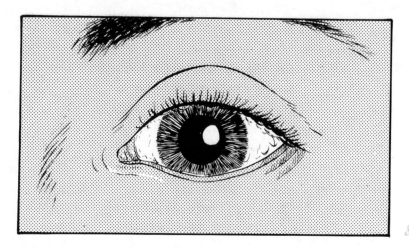

If your iris sits medium to high and you have medium to large eyes, then kohl pencil on the lower lid can assist in balancing the iris and creating a more defined look. If you have a medium-set iris then evening is a great time to apply kohl pencil, but it can look a little harsh during the day. If your eyes have a low-set iris, don't use kohl pencil.

As for kohl colours, I suggest charcoal, black or, in some cases, deep blue. Colours such as mauve, violet, brown or green can make the eyes look tired, so stay away from these.

To discover a simple way of applying kohl, see following.

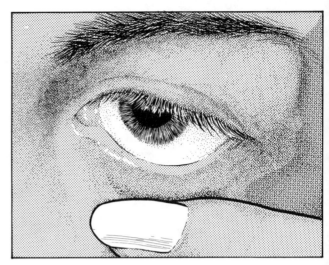

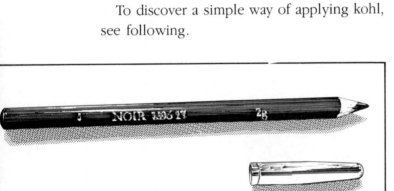

1 *Tools: Kohl pencil.*

2 *Tilt chin down and look up into mirror. Press under lower lid gently with finger. This helps lift the lower lid rim and makes it protrude slightly (don't pull the eye).*

3 *Now you can easily draw a steady line along the inside rim.*

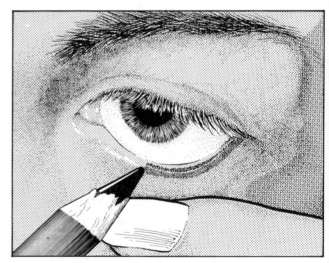

MASCARA

Here's a myth that, although not frequently spoken of, is being crystallised on the faces of thousands of women every day, especially those over 25. The myth goes like this: "It's alright to wear eyeshadow WITHOUT any mascara." Does this statement ring true to you?

Many women wear eyeshadow, but a large proportion of them don't apply mascara. If you do wear shadow without mascara, then there's a strong chance your eyes will take on a 'bald' appearance. The eyeshadow will coat the upper lashes and make them appear lighter. When the colour of your eyelashes fades, an ageing look can result.

For a natural, more youthful make-up, it is important to apply a little mascara. In fact, mascara is so important that I classify it as one of the three most basic make-up products for women over 25.

I spoke of 'feature-focusing' in an earlier chapter. Feature-focusing is the art of bringing your best features (eyes and mouth) forward so that any skin imperfections fade into the background. Mascara, lip pencil and lipstick are the three most basic of beneficial products in the art of feature-focusing. So, if you're really caught in a rush and only have time to apply a little make-up, you will benefit greatly from the three basics.

If you have an extra minute or two, add eyeliner to your lower lids and some brow colour. These products will bring your eyes and mouth forward, therefore softening any wrinkles, lines or imperfections.

If you feel a little uneasy about applying mascara, then it could be that you're concerned with one of the following points:

- You wear glasses and find it difficult to apply mascara.
- You're eyes are very sensitive to mascara.
- You find it difficult to keep your hand steady.

- Your mascara usually ends up all around your eye by the end of the day.

Well, let me see if I can give you some help with these problems.

- If you wear glasses or contacts or find it hard to see, then try a well-lit magnifying make-up mirror. They are excellent for helping you see your face in bright and even lighting. Use the 'daylight' setting to apply all your make-up, then check your finished make-up in the 'evening' light setting if required. (See A Clearer View, page 91).

- Sensitive eyes are a common problem. You should only purchase mascara especially made for sensitive eyes. Revlon make 'micropure'. Those from Clinique and Innoxa are also recommended.

- If you're having trouble holding your hand steady, you'll need to buy a mascara with a short wand. This will make it much easier for you to control the application of your mascara. Elizaben Arden make a good short-wand mascara called Two-Brush.

  Always keep a cotton bud handy for any little mistakes and try to use a hand mirror. Look up into it when doing lower lashes and down into it for upper lashes. (See application technique, pages 68-9).

- If your eyes resemble those of a racoon by the end of the day, then I think you'll need a waterproof mascara. If you do use one, make sure you have a good waterproof mascara remover to cleanse it off thoroughly each night.

An easy and effective way of enhancing your eyelashes without necessarily having to wear mascara would be to have them tinted. It's an option for those of you who'd really prefer not to wear mascara at all.

There are three common types of mascara: waterproof, lash-lengthening and water soluble. It's entirely up to you which of these is most suitable.

Waterproof is excellent in warmer climates as it tends not to smudge. The drawback is that unless you use it with a good eye make-up remover, it can be difficult to remove. Some lash-lengthening mascaras lengthen lashes by adding tiny fibres to the lashes. I don't like to use these, because the tiny fibres can break off and fall into your eyes. Be sure to check if the mascara contains fibres.

Water-soluble mascara seems to be quite popular as it's easy to remove and is also easy to apply.

What about the use of coloured mascara? Here's another myth: "Blue eyes look great with blue mascara."

Did you know that there are green, violet, aqua, white, blue and pink mascaras? The most popular of these are blue and violet.

Coloured mascaras such as these will do one particular thing for the wearer's eyes — they'll dominate! If you wear a bright blue mascara, what will people look at when they speak to you? Will they see into your eyes or will they stop at the bright blue eyelashes and fail to see your true beauty? You know the answer.

This book has been written to help you learn to create a natural, healthy and youthful make-up. Bright coloured mascaras don't fall into this category, so stay away from them. Black and dark brown are the best choices. I recommend dark brown only for a very fair complexion. If you have a mascara that is over six months old, please stop using it on your eyelashes. Go out and buy a fresh one, because bacteria breed quickly in opened mascaras, leading to the risk of eye infection.

Don't throw away your old mascara, keep it and see if you can use it for another purpose ... your eyebrows. Mascara on eyebrows? Curious? Then look at Eyebrows on pages 69-71 and see how you can effectively utilise your old dried-out mascara.

How to apply mascara ... see below.

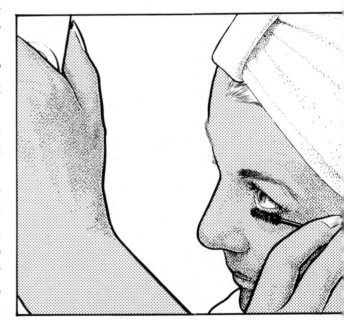

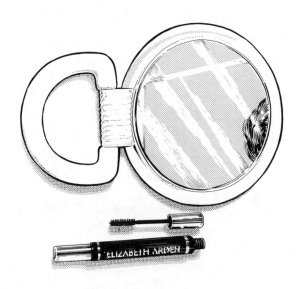

1 Tools: Mascara, hand mirror.

2 With mirror held high, tilt chin down and look up into mirror. (A hand mirror is best.) Now gently apply a coat of mascara firstly to the lower eye lashes.

3 With mirror held lower than your eye line, tilt your chin upwards and look down into mirror. Now apply a coat to the upper lashes.
Repeat both steps if you wish to add another coat of mascara.

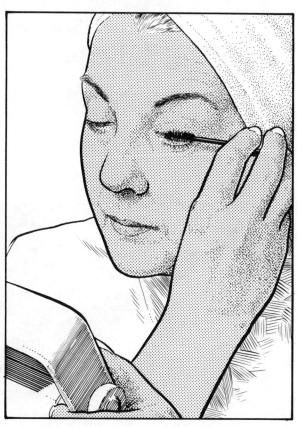

EYEBROWS

I'm not going to talk to you about changing your eyebrow shape. Surprised? I'm not even going to show you any clever diagrams on how to re-design your eyebrows totally, as you've no doubt seen it all before, anyway.

If you're over 25, you'll probably have a very 'stable' brow shape by now and I know that a radical fashion change to your eyebrow shape will definitely not make you look more naturally beautiful.

What I will tell you is that as you get older, your brows begin to fade and they can sometimes thin out, so you may need to give them some special attention.

It's important to note that your brows play a major role in creating facial balance, thus inviting attention to your eyes. They act as a frame for your eyes. The secret to 'ageless' brows is to keep them looking as natural as possible — that is, no hard lines.

I advise all women (especially if you wear eyeshadow) to have any fine, stray brow hairs growing under the brow line removed on a regular basis. If your brows tend to be a little long, then excess hairs can also be removed at the same time.

If you have trouble seeing these fine brow hairs, arrange to have them removed by a professional beauty therapist. It's quite inexpensive and the effect is most uplifting.

One thing I will share with you about eyebrow length is this: Don't let your eyebrow length be longer than one centimetre past the outer corner of your eye. If it is longer, you risk the look of 'drooping eyes' as the longer the brow, the older and heavier the eye looks. So, keep a check on the length.

Colouring your brows

I find that eyebrow tinting is an effective and inexpensive way of colouring your brows and only needs to be repeated every few weeks. If you have difficulty colouring your eyebrows, eyebrow tinting is worth a try.

Throw away your eyebrow pencils

That's right, eyebrow pencils are one of the most harsh and ageing of all make-up products sold today. More money saved! They're great for the stage, but how often are you on stage?

If your brows need colour, then here's an old product and a new technique for you. It's far more natural and flattering. Take a mascara

1 Tools: Old or dried-out mascara, a brow brush, tissue.

2 If mascara is not dry enough, wipe excess from wand onto tissue.

3 Carefully brush (don't press) up all along your brow line. This requires practice as only a light coat of colour should be deposited onto the brows.

4 Use a brow brush to brush gently over brows and remove excess colour.

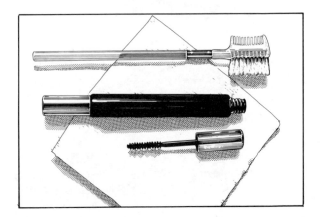

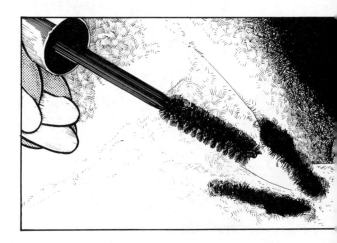

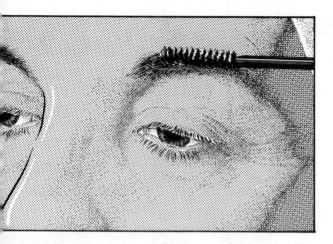

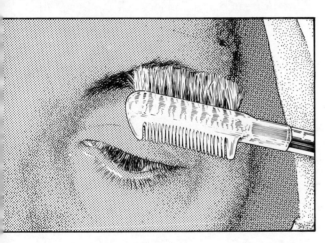

What about bald patches that may occur in eyebrows? A brow powder, such as Revlon's Brow Beautiful, does a great job of filling in any eyebrow gaps and the mascara will give you the fullness you need.

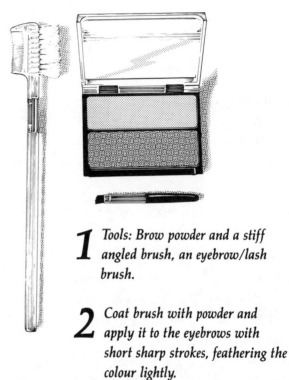

1 *Tools: Brow powder and a stiff angled brush, an eyebrow/lash brush.*

2 *Coat brush with powder and apply it to the eyebrows with short sharp strokes, feathering the colour lightly.*

(preferably an old, dried-up one) and gently run it upwards through your brow hairs, all the way along your brow line.

You can use brown, dark brown or black mascara. Make sure the mascara is dry and not moist and gluggy. If you don't have an old, dry mascara, then buy a cheap one, open it and leave it open for a day or so until it dries out. If you have a fairly moist mascara, wipe off the excess on the wand with a tissue.

This is a wonderful way of feature-focusing your eyebrows. It looks much more natural.

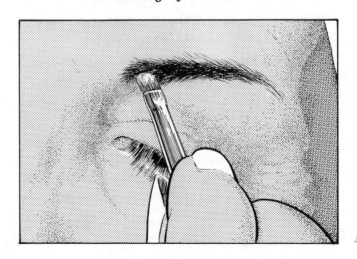

Foundation

harmonise your skin tone

*H*ave you ever stopped to think why we wear foundation? What is it supposed to do? The two major reasons for introducing foundation base are:

- To even out the colour in the face (skin tone).

- To act as a 'base coat' for improved application of any other make-up products after the foundation.

I'd like to ask what type of 'coverage' you'd like. Do you like a natural sheer look, or perhaps, a surer coverage which eliminates any skin discoloration?

Before you purchase a foundation base, be aware of exactly how much coverage you want. I suggest that as you get older it's best to keep your foundation looking fairly natural. Remember, feature-focusing your make-up is the aim, and heavy foundations only highlight lines and wrinkles. Avoid them.

There are many types of foundation and the art of selection can be very confusing. Among these are water-based, oil-free and oil-based foundations. The water-based types include the following: cake make-up, mousse, and creams which contain a little oil and are suitable for all skin types as they give a light to medium coverage. I recommend these because they look more natural.

If you need a heavier coverage, an oil-based foundation such as a panstick will be best. Oil-free foundations are especially formulated for women with oily skin and while they may assist in controlling an oily look, they can be difficult to apply.

The best way to be sure of achieving the coverage you want is to actually try the tester foundation first before you purchase it. Before I lead into colour, I'd like to explain that wearing foundation base is often more likely to protect your skin from the ageing effects of the environment than pollute it. So, if you haven't worn foundation because you thought it would clog your pores, this should be welcome news. Always use a good make-up remover. For more on cleansing and preparing your skin for make-up see page 89.

How do you choose the best colour? The most important factor in searching for the correct shade of foundation base is to match it as closely as possible to your own skin colour (on the face).

Once you know which type of coverage you like, then it's time to choose the ideal colour. The best way to do this is to try the tester on your face. (See the foundation application illustrations below and on the following page.) Select two or three foundation colours and place them on your face side by side (along your jaw). Wait a few minutes to decide which of the shades most resembles your skin colour.

Don't try the foundation on your wrist, neck or back of your hand as the skin colour on these areas differs from that on your face.

When checking for foundation colours make sure you're in natural (not incandescent) light so that you can clearly see the true colours.

Have you ever been tempted to buy a 'summer' foundation (one darker than your own skin tone) for the illusion of a healthy tan?

Don't! Avoid these especially if you are over 25, because a foundation darker than your own skin colour will age you. If you want to look naturally attractive, keep the foundation you use as close as possible to the colour of your own face.

See the following instructions for a detailed description of how best to apply your foundation.

Here's a foundation myth:

1   If you have a ruddy (red) complexion, use a yellow (warm) toned foundation to counteract your ruddiness.

2   If you have a sallow (yellow) complexion use a pink (cool) toned foundation to counteract your sallowness.

1   Tools: Foundation base, latex sponge, spatula (to remove foundation base).

2   Dot foundation over face, making sure that the centre of face (nose, chin area) has a little extra coverage.

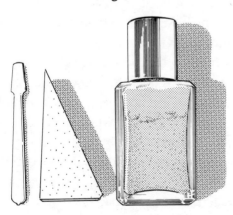

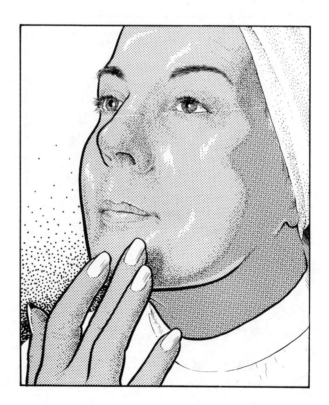

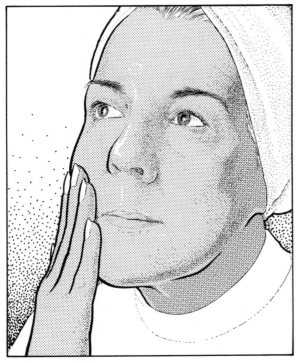

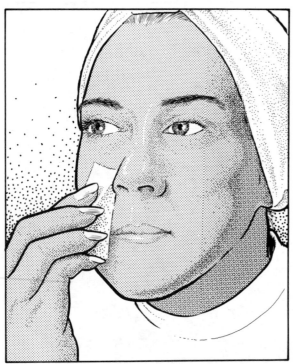

3 *Firmly and briskly pat in foundation base, gradually thinning it out toward your hair and jawlines. (Ensure that you have no demarcation line along your jaw. It should look natural.)*

4 *For an even, blended look, use your latex sponge to press and roll the foundation. This assists blending and absorbs excess foundation. (You can use your sponge either dry or damp.)*

I don't know about you, but I've been told the above many times in the past by qualified cosmetic salespeople. The worst thing of all is that the theory sounded logical, but, in practice, it could become the basis of a disastrously unnatural-looking make-up.

Your skin colour will eventually show through and the effect will be a blotchy mess of oranges and pinks.

If you do have either a ruddy or sallow complexion, resist the temptation to alter it drastically. It's best to select a foundation colour that harmonises with that of your skin, and use the best eye make-up and lip colours to feature-focus your make-up. This will then detract from an overpowering skin tone.

What about concealer? Concealer is designed to minimise dark areas such as pimples, smile lines and so on. While a good, heavy concealer will mask these imperfections, your face would probably 'crack' if you dared to smile or laugh. Many of the coversticks (concealers) you buy today are very heavy and unnatural, not at all the ingredient for youthful, natural looking make-up. If you follow the directions in this book, namely those on feature-focusing, you will find that theatrical concealers won't be necessary.

The only concealer I recommend for everyday wear is the wand type, not the stick type (which is heavy). A good natural looking one is Amway's automatic concealer. If you do have dark circles under your eyes, a touch of concealer will definitely help. But try not to use it on deep facial lines as it will tend to 'crack' and make the lines more prominent.

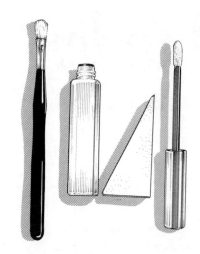

As for concealer colour, go for a shade which is a little lighter than your own skin (but not too much so). For very dark circles, try a concealer which is identical to the colour of your skin. When you apply concealer under your eyes, make sure you blend it only on the inner half of your eye. If you apply it to the outer corners of your eye, you will only highlight any lines or wrinkles and make the eye look puffy.

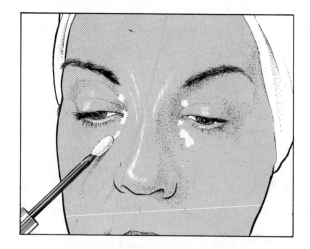

To find out how best to apply concealer see the following illustrations.

1 Tools: Wand type concealer, latex wedge sponge, eyeshadow brush (for hard to get to areas).

2 Dot concealer on lower inner corner of eye and if required along the upper inner corner of your eye. (For deep shadow area only.)

3 Blend by patting with fingertip, a small brush or corner of sponge.

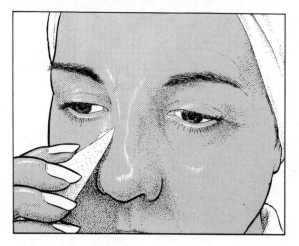

Powder

a natural look

*I*f you're using a liquid, mousse or creme foundation, a little loose powder is necessary. It will assist in giving the foundation a matt appearance and offer a little extra life to your make-up.

The most widely used powder is translucent; that is, a no-colour powder. For a natural looking make-up, I suggest translucent loose powder for your initial make-up. If you need to touch-up your make-up during the day, compact or pressed translucent powders are available. For those of you with darker skin tones, shop around for powder that's closer to the colour of your skin for a more natural look. (See the section on recommendations for dark skins, page 92.)

Now, for instructions on powder application see the following illustrations.

1 *Tools: Powder brush or powder puff, loose powder.*

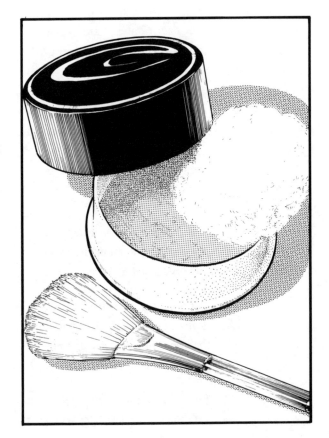

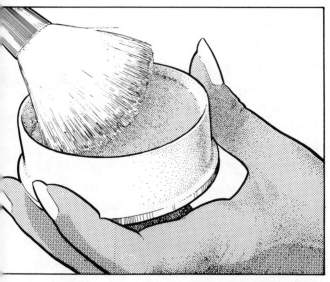

2 *After applying foundation base, coat your powder brush with loose powder. Now dust off excess powder on the back of your hand before applying to your face.*

3 *Dust powder brush down face with a little extra coverage across nose and chin area. If you intend to apply eyeshadow, then dust a little powder over lid area also. If using a powder puff, simply coat puff lightly with powder and press all over face. To remove excess, dust face well with clean powder brush.*

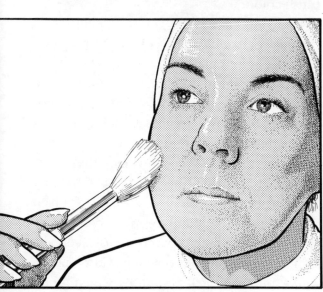

Blush
enhance your natural tone

*H*ere's another myth you may have heard before: "You must always select your blush colour to co-ordinate exactly with your clothes colour."

Blush is not to be used as a fashion accessory. Its major role is to enhance your natural skin tone; its supporting role is to be compatible with your clothing colour.

Have you also heard that blush can be used as a contour or shader, especially if placed on chin, jawline or the tip of your nose? It's been widely claimed that the placement of blush on the above areas will give your face a 'lift', or better still, help to conceal any imperfections.

Wrong! Blush is a colour that should be applied to the cheek area to enhance the natural skin tone. It should not be used as a concealer or magical lift to eradicate so-called facial flaws. In fact, blush applied to your chin, jawline and nose in order to conceal will only attract further attention to these areas.

NOTE: *There is some confusion concerning the use of blush as a shader (contour). The use of shader is explained in* Evening Tricks.

Blush colour

Now you know blush is not to be used as a fashion accessory and that it's primary purpose is one of enhancing your natural skin tone, you must be wondering why on earth there are so many different blush colours available on the market.

I believe that, like eyeshadows, most of these shades are a sales ploy and, therefore, a waste of money. Many of the available blush shades fall into the ageing, useless or frosted colour category, just like eyeshadows. (Doesn't this make it so much simpler to find your best blush colour?)

Knowing that what you're seeking is a natural, compatible blush colour, I've prepared a simple colour chart illustrating two colours to enhance most skins. Remember, these colours must be matt, not frosted (sparkling); a frosted blush will accentuate lines, wrinkles or small imperfections in the skin.

If you're not certain which of these two shades of blush will be the most enhancing for you, then try this test. First ask yourself which lipstick colours are your best: those from the warm range (peaches, rusts, coppers etc) or those from the cool range (burgundies, pinks, plums etc)? If you know which group is the most flattering for you, then you can select either the warmer toned blush or the cooler blush shade.

Another alternative, if you're still confused, is to remove the coloured blush swatches from the chart and hold these up to your face while you look into a well-lit mirror. Turn away and look back again, repeating the process until you realise which blush colour most harmonises with your face (the one that doesn't clash). This will be your best colour.

Which blush: powder or creme? This is a question often asked, especially by the over twenty-fives. I find powder blush to be the easiest and most effective, but creme blush works well in some cases, such as for women with extremely long, thin faces, pigmentation (brown marks or freckles) or very dry, flaky skin. Creme blush can give the skin a natural, translucent glow, although it's not recommended for oily or acne-prone skin.

And now for the next myth to be exploded: "The application of your blush depends on which of the seven basic face shapes you possess."

This theory is long outdated and not at all relevant for you in this real life, away from TV/cameras and theatre stages.

What I've created on page 42 are the two new face shapes; they're simple to follow. First, determine in which category you belong. Look directly into your mirror and see if you have a narrow or wide face.

These two diagrams show you where to apply your blush. Look to see which of the two is closest to your face size. If your face is a combination of the two, your blush application will also be a combination of both narrow and wide.

For a precise explanation on how to apply your blush, look at the illustrations that follow.

See the blush colours in the Natural Compatible Colours chart on page 34 for the best colour recommendations.

Above all else, remember to use your blush to enhance your natural skin tone and not to overpower it.

NOTE: *This sequence is targeted specifically to those with little or no blush 'placement' experience.*

1 Tools: Blush, tissue, small blush brush, latex wedge sponge.

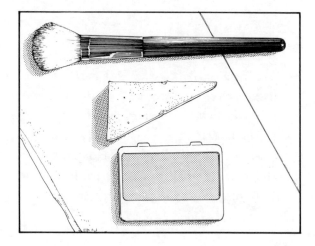

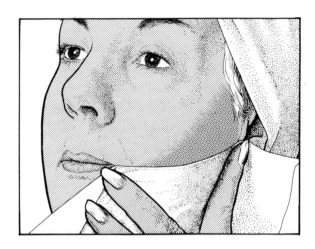

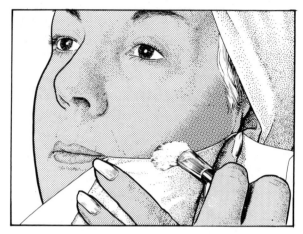

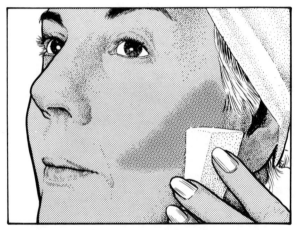

2 Hold a folded tissue neatly in a line between your lower ear and the corner of your mouth.

3 Coat your brush well with blush (always dust off excess on back of your hand) and apply to tissue in upward strokes, overlapping at least 4 centimetres or 1½ inches onto your cheek area. Brush upwards all along tissue, as evenly as possible, from ear inward and back again (don't go beyond vertical dotted lines on blush diagrams).

4 Remove tissue and with corner of sponge blend harsh blush line in downward strokes, until well blended. Press your sponge all over blush area until it looks natural. If you require more blush, simply add a little more and blend carefully. Once you feel confident about applying your blush, begin again without the tissue. The tissue method is really for beginners.

NOTE: *If you have already applied shader (see Evening Tricks, page 94) with the tissue method, you may wish to eliminate using the tissue method again with your blush. In this case, simply apply your blush over the shader, from ear towards nose area. (Do not go past dotted line.) Bend carefully with your latex sponge.*

Lip Pencil
breaking the age barrier

Yes, that's right! A lip pencil used correctly can make you look younger by detracting from lines, wrinkles and other so-called facial imperfections.

As your face gets older, your lip colour and lip contour tend to fade. Another frequent occurrence is the appearance of vertical lines forming through the lip line itself. These tiny lines play havoc with your lipstick, (especially if you don't use a lip pencil). The lipstick creeps or bleeds through these lines, outside your original lip line, and gives your lipstick a feathered effect.

If you want to feature-focus your make-up, lip pencil will work wonders. By re-defining your lips with pencil it will effectively give the impression of bringing your lips forward. In other words, the lip pencil will clearly define your lips and in so doing will automatically detract from any imperfections.

1 *Tools: Lip pencil (outline), cotton bud (for mistakes).*

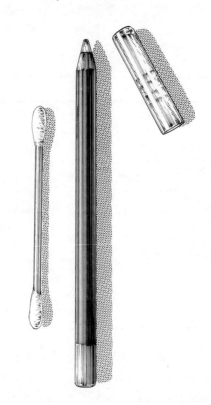

NOTE: *Hold the pencil close to the tip and lean your little finger on your chin for added support.*

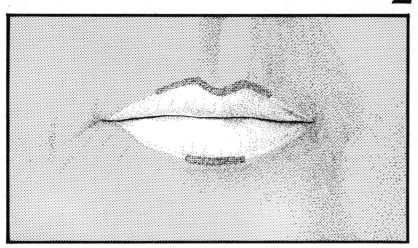

2 Begin by outlining your cupid's bow. Many of you will find that you have either a lop-sided cupid's bow or you seem to have none to speak of. Rest assured that we are the majority and not the minority!

The secret to great looking lips is practice! Practice, that is, at balancing up an uneven lip line. Firstly decide which side of your lips (left or right) you like best (usually the fuller side) and outline this part of the cupid's bow firmly. Next step is to match the other side, even if it means straightening it up to look like your best side. The general idea is to create a 'balanced' lip line, so a little cheating is alright.

The next step is to line the centre of your bottom lip (about one centimetre/¹⁄₃ inch).

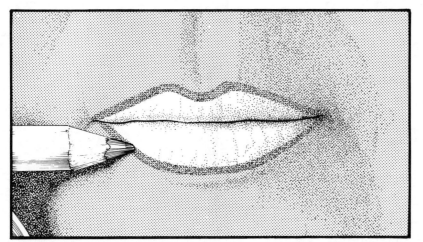

3 Here's the tricky part. This is where you need practice! Begin to join the lines and try to match the left side to the right. Select your best side and duplicate this on the other side. Try not to over-exaggerate your lip line as all we want to accomplish is an even, natural-looking outline.

If you decide to use a lip fill-in pencil, you may want to thicken your darker outlining pencil. This is especially beneficial for those of you with uneven lip lines. You will achieve a great natural look once you've blended in the 'fill-in' pencil later.

The Balancing Act
eyes and lips

*L*ine your lips before you apply eye make-up. You've probably never heard this before, have you? That's because this book is a first in explaining make-up from an artistic perspective.

A basic key to art is balance. In an earlier chapter, I said that the features most noticed were your eyes and mouth. If these two features appear out of balance, then you'll risk looking unnatural and, possibly, tired or older.

The best way to ensure balance between your eye make-up and your lips is to outline your lips with lip pencil before applying eye make-up. (Don't apply lipstick until last). Try it, you'll be surprised by how much easier it will be to apply your eye make-up. Using this technique, you'll be able to use your lipline as a reference point as often as you like, while doing your eyes.

Durable lipstick: the secret

The secret of durable lipstick lies in the use of a 'fill-in' lip pencil. This should be a colour which is pale and almost identical to your natural lip colour. (Try Revlon's 'nude' pencil or Yves Rocher 'naturelle'). If you have darker lips, you may have to search for a natural shade which is closer in colour to your natural lip tone.

Try the durable lipstick technique. After outlining your lips with a deep shade, fill in the entire lip area with a paler, fill-in pencil, while making sure to blend it a little with the deeper outline. (This helps to soften the hard edge). This technique works well and helps to stop lipstick from bleeding.

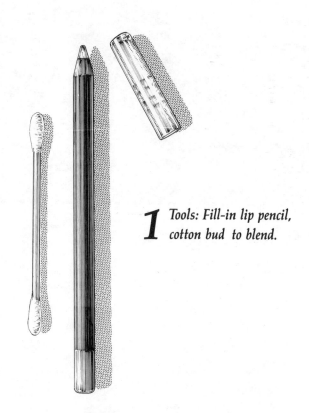

1 *Tools: Fill-in lip pencil, cotton bud to blend.*

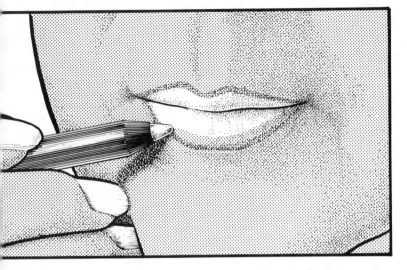

2 *Once you've outlined your lips with a darker outlining pencil, you can begin to fill-in with this natural lip-coloured pencil. (This really helps to keep lipstick on longer.)*
Try to overlap your fill-in pencil with the harder edges of the outline pencil first. A muted, blended effect is far more attractive than leaving a harsh lip outline.

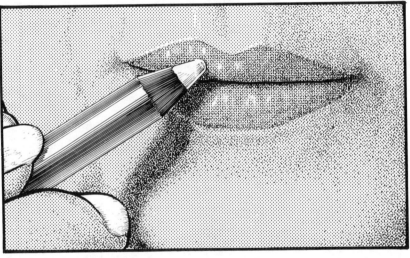

3 *Fill in remainder of lip area with your pencil.*

Changing your lip shape

You won't see the usual diagrams depicting ways of shortening, lengthening, reducing or enlarging your lips in this book. Those special techniques are best reserved for theatre, photographic or film work, where special effects lighting and touch-up work are utilised.

For everyday wear, keep your mouth shape as close to your natural line as possible.

Because most of us have an uneven lipline, always begin lining your lips in the centre. See the diagram on lip-lining, page 82.

If you make a mistake in your lip-lining, simply wipe it off, wiping inwards towards the centre of your mouth, and then start again (use a cotton bud).

If you're a bit shaky or if you've had little experience at lip-lining, don't give up, please. Hold your pencil as close to the tip as possible and lean your little finger on your chin. This will give you some stability. Don't get disheartened if you slip and find the pencil line nearer to your nose than your lips. We all started somewhere.

The following is another make-up myth! "Buy a separate lip pencil for each of your different lipstick colours."

This is crazy. If you have a fetish for lipstick pencils, that's fine, but if not, then you only need one or two outlining colours for all your lipsticks. For all burgundy, pink and plum lipsticks, use a deep plum or burgundy pencil

(such as Revlon's Plum). For all terracotta, rust, peach and orange lipsticks, use a deep terracotta (Helena Rubinstein's Raisin).

Because you're feature-focusing your mouth, you need to use a 'defining' colour on your lip line. It must be a 'deep' colour to outline and define your mouth. A medium to pale lip line will only blur your mouth and make your lips appear older. Remember that if you use the fill-in pencil technique, then this pale colour will soften the effect of the dark lip line.

Later, after applying your lipstick, look closely to see that your lip line is not showing through too harshly. It should be muted.

A factor usually overlooked, but essential to a great-looking lip line, is the use of a sharp pencil. Only a sharpened lip pencil will give you the definition you want. Inexpensive cosmetic sharpeners can be purchased at major department stores.

Lipstick

a feature focus

Did you know that there are ageing colours in lipstick, just as there are in blush and eyeshadow?

Some lipstick shades are ageing and lifeless while others lift your features and give a more natural, youthful glow. These more youthful lipstick shades I've named the Natural Compatible Colours, while ageing colours I've named the 'decorative colours', because, like blue and green eyeshadow, these lipstick shades detract from the beauty of your features by overpowering them. They're pretty colours to look at in themselves but do little or nothing to enhance your lips.

The least complimentary of all lipstick shades are mauves, purples and pale oranges. These are ageing colours.

While I'm on the subject of ageing colours, avoid wearing pale, pale lipsticks or heavily frosted ones. They'll make you look ill, tired and/or older. As I said in the lip pencil chapter, to achieve great-looking lips, the lips need to be defined to bring them forward (feature-focusing), but the application of a pale or heavily frosted lipstick will achieve the opposite result.

Lightly pearlised lipsticks are tolerable, but creme lipsticks tend to be more naturally attractive as you get older. I've found that most of us wear lipsticks with which we feel safe; that is, we select either pale, medium, vivid or deep tones of lipsticks.

I think that as you get older it's best to select from the medium to vivid shades of lipstick. Pale, pale is out and very deep coloured lipsticks can make your mouth look vamp-ish or vampire-ish!

As for a foolproof way to select your perfect lipstick colour, I have to admit that I haven't found one. However, a technique that I've found quite successful is to select several lipstick shades that you are attracted to, one group belonging to the warm shades (peaches, rusts, coppers, etc), and one group belonging to the cool shades (burgundies, pinks, plums, etc). Now look into your well-lit mirror and hold the group of warm lipsticks up to your mouth. Look at your face and turn away, and then repeat the step. The lipstick shade which dominates your face will usually be your least attractive alternative. This should then leave you with the most harmonising shades.

You may find that none of the warmer shades of lipstick are flattering, which may indicate the cool tones would be more attractive for you. If this is the case, repeat the selection process, only this time with the cool toned lipsticks, until you have found the ones that you like.

To assist you in your search for lipsticks that make you look younger, healthier and more natural, I've prepared a lipstick colour chart (the Natural Compatible Colours, page 34) illustrating nine of the best possible shades. If the lipsticks themselves are not available to try, then you could remove each colour and hold it up to your face as recommended previously.

What about changing your lip shape? No! Redesigning your lip shape is out for everyday wear. Turn to page 84 and I'll explain why (see changing your lip shape).

Are there longer-lasting lipstick formulae? Yes, look for lipsticks which feel drier when you apply them. They lack the glossed look of more moisturising lipsticks, but they stay on longer. Glossy lipsticks, because they are more moist, tend to melt and bleed. If you have small or thin lips then glossy lipsticks are definitely a no-no for you.

When should you use a lip brush? There are two major reasons for using a lip brush:

1 A lip brush ensures a more even application; in other words, it's easier to keep your lipstick from smudging outside your lipline.

2 You're able to apply more of the lipstick colour, therefore achieving a longer-lasting application.

If you have medium to small lips, a lip brush will give you a precision application. It's a necessity for all women with small lips. However, if your lips are large, you may well be able to apply lipstick without using a brush and still achieve a professional effect. For correct lipstick application steps, see the illustrations on page 88.

Remember, whatever size your lips may be, always use a lip pencil before applying lipstick.

1 *Tools: Lip brush, lipstick.*

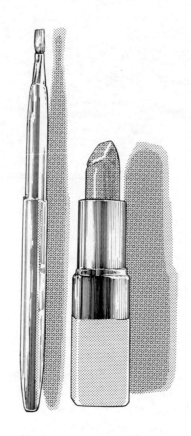

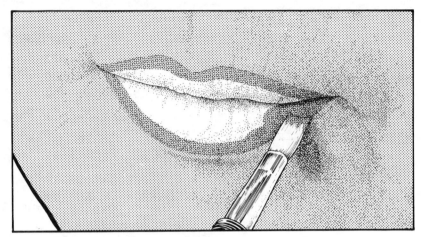

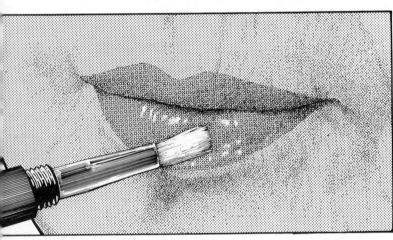

2 *Coat your lip brush well with lipstick and try to follow your lip line as close to the edge as possible.*

3 *Now you can fill remaining lip area with lipstick.*

Sun-Block

preparing for make-up

We have now entered the time where applying a sun-block has become a necessity. With the ozone layer deteriorating, the sun's more harmful rays can penetrate and damage the skin quite severely. If you wish to protect your skin from both cancer and ageing, you will need to apply at least a SPF15 (sun protection factor) sun-block every day.

Which goes on first, sun-block or moisturiser? If you use both, apply your sun-block before your moisturiser, but wait 10-20 minutes in between application. Ideally, a sun-block (SPF15) with a built-in moisturiser would save time.

When you purchase a sun-block cream for your face, preferably select one that is transparent and non-greasy. Watch out for skin sensitivity too, as sometimes the waterproof formulae can irritate your skin.

Cleansing routine

Contrary to all the fuss and confusion within the cosmetic industry about what is best for your face, I believe in keeping things simple and inexpensive.

A good daily cleansing routine with a little moisturiser and sun-block are all you really need to prepare the skin for make-up. It's simple and it works. Keeping a clean face is the most important factor.

If you have patchy, dry or scaly skin and it feels like sandpaper, you may well need to remove the surface dead skin cell layer. Contact a professional beauty therapist and ask for a mild facial peel or use a good skin buffing creme yourself at home. Buffing your skin will improve circulation and remove surface dead skin cells, leaving your skin smooth for applying make-up. Always check the product ingredients and seek professional advice if you have sensitive skin.

Another common problem is dry lips or having fine feather lines. I recommend using Elizabeth Arden's Lip-Fix creme. Use a little on and around your lips before application, it keeps your lips from drying out.

To ensure healthy, clean skin you also need to have a good procedure for taking off your make-up. Even if you use only a moderate amount of make-up, use a good eye make-up remover. I recommend Yves Rocher eye make-up remover gel and Revlon's eye make-up remover gel. Be sure to rinse your face and eyes well after cleansing.

If you wish to learn more about skin care, get a copy of *Blue eyeshadow should still be illegal* by Paul Begoun (Beginning Press).

7-minute Make-up

super-quick that lasts all day

If you only have five to seven minutes to apply your make-up, but you'd like it to last all day, here is a six-step make-up technique that will feature-focus your face while still looking natural.

Simply follow the instructions and turn to each illustrated step as you go. Make sure you've selected your best colours first.

1 *FOUNDATION AND POWDER*
(see pages 73-4 and 76-7)

2 *LIP PENCIL*
(see page 82)

3 *BLUSH*
(see page 80)

4 *EYELINER*
(see pages 62-3)

5 *MASCARA*
(see pages 68-9)

6 *LIPSTICK*
(see page 88)

A Clearer View
lighting and magnification

One of the most important and yet most neglected factors in achieving a good make-up is lighting. Have you ever had to apply your make-up in a dimly lit room, or experienced lop-sided lighting? This usually leaves you wondering all day if your face looks crooked.

Do a lighting check in the room in which you apply your make-up. Is it adequate? Are there windows on both sides, giving you equal light? Or do you have one single light above the mirror, thereby casting hollow shadows on your face?

If you're serious about making your make-up job easier, faster and more appealing, think about improving your present lighting situation if that's a problem.

Apart from having good, natural and even daylight, here are two suggestions.

◢ Buy a portable (electric) make-up mirror (right), using the strongest light setting to apply your make-up; or

◢ Attach non-incandescent or fluorescent lights to both sides of your bathroom or bedroom mirror.

Incandescent lighting is often too flattering and make-up mistakes are difficult to detect in this type of lighting.

If you have eyesight problems, a professional, portable, double-sided make-up mirror is probably the best for you. You need one with a large magnifying mirror and a strong light setting to illuminate your face well. When applying make-up to areas such as eyes and lips, you'll need to see even closer. Buy a small magnifying hand mirror and hold this close with one hand, while you do your finer, more controlled brush strokes with the other.

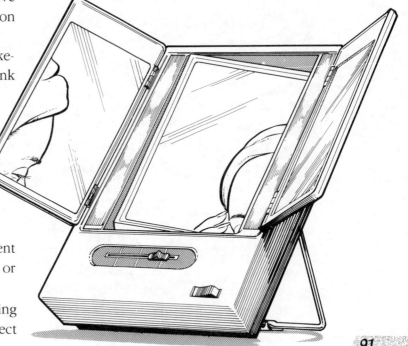

Dark skin
make-up recommendations

*I*f you have dark skin, there is only one variation from all the principles and teachings I have set out in this book.

The principles of balance, light and shade still apply. However, in the area of colour, you'll need to note the following:

- Stay away from paler shades of make-up as these will only make you appear washed-out.

- Your lipstick, blush and eyeshadow colour need to be more intense for them to do a good job of feature-focusing.

- Select a foundation shade as close to your skin colour as possible. Use a powder to set the foundation and remove excess shine. The powder shade should also be close to your skin colour.

- Although some of you may be able to get away successfully with blue or green eyeshadows, these colours tend to dominate rather than enhance the natural beauty of your eyes. For an example, see Lorna, Plate 13, page 31. Lorna is wearing green eyeshadow. It appears lifeless, whereas you'll see her eyes light up in corals and violet shadows in Plate 14.

- For some interesting eyeshadow combinations, see the Eyeshadow Combination Chart on pages 28-9. Experiment with any of the combinations, but try to avoid the paler light and deep colours. Select the more vivid, intense eyeshadow colours.

- As for blush, you'll need to go for intensity of colour to lift out the colour of your cheeks.

- Lipstick shades may be tricky, as frosted lipsticks can exaggerate your lips and make them appear puffy. If you have a darker skin tone, you can wear deeper and more vivid shades of lipstick. Experiment to find the shades with which you feel comfortable. Look at the lipstick chart, the Natural Compatible Colours on page 34.

Blemishes
scars & birthmarks

*I*f you have a facial imperfection that you'd like to conceal (ie scar, birthmark or pigmentation), the easiest way to do this is to purchase a concealing foundation base to disguise the area.

Because of the difficulty you may have in finding the one 'perfect' shade to do the job, you will probably need to buy two shades of foundation base and mix them so that the colour appears more natural.

There are many products available that are specifically designed to conceal scars, birthmarks or pigmentation. Two brand names I can recommend to you are Kryolan and Dermablend foundations. These bases are quite heavy and consequently give an excellent coverage.

Once you have selected your foundation, take particular care to read instructions on its application. It's a good idea to ask the sales consultant to show you exactly how to apply your foundation so that it gives a look that is as natural as possible.

If you do have a problem with scars, birthmarks and pigmentation, try to focus on the positive areas of your face rather than expending too much energy, product or money trying to cover your so-called imperfection. Remember, you are beautiful ...

Evening Tricks
a softer light

What do you think the basic differences would be between a day and evening make-up? Believe it or not, evening make-up need only be a more intense form of day make-up. Don't think that because it's night time you can get away with all the little theatrical shading tricks I've been trying to talk you out of.

Some of you may be proficient at minimal shading of areas such as double chins and wide noses, but whether it's a day or evening make-up, 'feature-focusing' not facial shading, is the real key to a successful make-up.

The biggest difference between your day and evening make-up will be the lighting. Evening light is usually much softer than daylight, so a more pronounced make-up is required. Consequently there are a few additions you may like to include in your evening make-up.

The first area is foundation base. It's a good idea to apply either a foundation with a little heavier coverage or apply a second coat of your usual day base. Don't forget a little powder to stop shine. (See foundation application steps, pages 72-3).

The second area which you may or may not wish to include is the subtle shading of your cheek socket area. This area is the only 'shading' area I believe is occasionally necessary for a great evening make-up. Deepening or shading inside your cheek hollow creates the illusion of bringing your cheek area forward. You will need to buy a powder shader (no frost) such as Revlon's Brow Beautiful in dark brown. Although intended for the brows, it can be used sparingly on your cheek socket.

A good quality small blush brush is great for applying the shader. If you wish to experiment with this effect, see the following illustrations. Good luck! (If you have a narrow face, eliminate this step as it could accentuate the narrowness.)

Third, eye make-up can be defined more for evening by lining your upper lid with black or charcoal. This gives the illusion that your eyelashes are much thicker. For large eyes or eyes with a high-set iris, a little kohl pencil inside the lower lid adds definition. As for special combinations of eyeshadow and eyeliner colours, see the Eyeshadow Combination Chart on pages 28-9 and the Eyeliner Colour Combination Chart on pages 30-1.

For evening, you can add a little more of your deeper shade of eyeshadow, and don't forget your eyebrows.

Last but not least, evening is a great time

for applying either a brighter or deeper shade of lipstick than you may normally wear during the day. Experiment if you can.

Here's a hint if you're wearing a red outfit, but can't wear red lipstick. Select a lipstick that is fairly neutral (not hot pink or bright orange) that you can wear well. Find a 'red' lipstick, scrape a little off and mix it with your wearable lipstick. Now apply it to your lips. This way your lipstick won't clash with your red outfit and it certainly won't clash with your face, either. (See lip pencil application on pages 81-2 and lipstick application on page 88.)

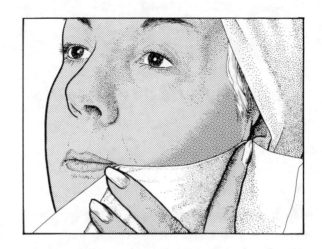

1 *Use after foundation and powder. Hold a folded tissue neatly in a line between the lower ear and the corner of your mouth.*

2 *Coat your blush brush with powder shader and apply to tissue in an upwards movement, making sure the shader overlaps onto skin by about 2½ centimetres (one inch). Go evenly all along tissue then back again towards ear.*

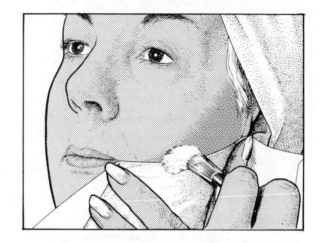

3 *Remove tissue. Holding latex wedge sponge, firmly and gently blend the hard shader edge in downward strokes until it's well blended. Now apply blush.*

NOTE: *Keep shader behind dotted line — do not shade near centre of face.*

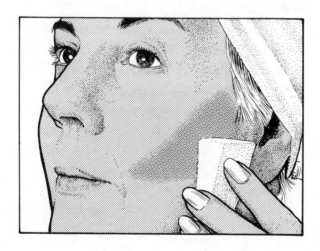

Brushes
choosing the right tools

You will find it almost impossible to create a great looking make-up without using the correct brushes. In fact, applying your make-up with shabby brushes or foam applicators (like the ones sold in eyeshadow compacts) will give you a theatrical, messy or streaky looking make-up. Another problem will arise with blending, as it is very difficult to blend when using the incorrect tools. If you want a natural, durable make-up, the appropriate brushes for blush, eyeshadow and lipstick are essential.

Look carefully at the illustrations (the tools for each make-up product sequence) and make sure when you do your purchasing that you match your brush heads to them both in shape and size.

Don't be tempted to use the foam eyeshadow applicators or the large-style blush brushes. If you have a look at the photos of the models in this book you will see clearly the results of using incorrect brushes and tools in the 'incorrect' make-up shots. You will see a remarkable difference in the 'correct' shots. See how well the eyeshadow and blush have been blended? That is the result of using the ideal shape and size of brush. These essential tools need not be expensive. The Princess range of brushes is acceptable and quite inexpensive.

Now, let's talk about how to use these brushes. First, never press the brush too firmly into your chosen colour. Just gently stroke your brush along it, then dust off the excess (you can do this on the back of your hand). It is vital that you do this so that you don't apply a big splash of colour to one small area, thus making it difficult to blend.

Practice makes perfect

Here's some good news! After teaching the principles in this book to over 4500 women, the 'success' rate feedback has been wonderful. These women are now able to apply a more beautiful and naturally attractive make-up, while spending far less on make-up purchases. In other words, they know exactly what to buy and where and how to apply it.

Most of the women I've taught are over 25 years old and many of them wear either contact lenses or glasses. The one thing that nearly all of them had in common was their initial fear of trying a new make-up technique. Some had shaky hands, some had eyesight problems, while most had hardly any artistic experience when it came to working on their eye make-up with professional brushes.

Most of these women overcame their initial fear within their first practice, saying it was much easier than they had imagined it would be. After two or three full make-up practices, they were feeling quite confident.

You may find make-up application to certain areas more difficult than others. All you need to do is practise. The first time you tried to ride a bicycle or drive a car, it all seemed well nigh impossible. Practice was the key, as it is with all new learning experiences. If everyone stopped learning how to drive because of their initial fear, we wouldn't get very far, would we? All you have to do with your make-up is try. That's it, have a go!

Of all the make-up application areas, my research has shown that eye make-up and use of the lip pencil seem to need the most practice. All I can advise is that you find the area you have the most difficulty with and set a couple of hours aside to work on it exclusively, until you feel confident. Apply the make-up, cleanse it off and re-apply it again. (Remember to always apply foundation base under eyeshadow if you're doing your eyes.)

If you have a problem with your eyesight or perhaps are having difficulty with the lighting, see A Clearer View on page 91.

Practise all you like, because eventually you'll not only have a fantastic make-up but you'll find you've applied it in 10 minutes or less!

Obtaining Your Natural Compatible Colours

For further information about where to obtain the natural compatible make-up colours used and recommended in this book, write to:

Nouk Tayler-Vieira
Natural Compatibles by Nouk
PO Box 22
Earlville
Cairns Qld 4870
Australia